Worksite Health Promotion

David H. Chenoweth, PhD, FAWHP

East Carolina University, Greenville, North Carolina
President, Health Management Associates
New Bern, North Carolina

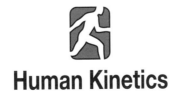

Human Kinetics

Library of Congress Cataloging-in-Publication Data

Chenoweth, David H., 1952-
    Worksite health promotion / by David H. Chenoweth.
      p. cm.
    Includes bibliographical references and index.
    ISBN 0-88011-542-4
    1. Health promotion. 2. Industrial hygiene. I. Title.
  RC969.H43C484   1998   97-39341
  658.3'82--dc21   CIP

ISBN: 0-88011-542-4

Acquisitions Editor: Scott Wikgren; **Developmental Editor:** Elaine Mustain; **Assistant Editors:** Melinda Graham, Cassandra Mitchell, and John Wentworth; **Copyeditor:** John Wentworth; **Proofreader:** Myla Smith; **Indexer:** Gerry Lynn Messner; **Graphic Designer:** Stuart Cartwright; **Graphic Artist:** Yvonne Winsor; **Photo Editor:** Boyd LaFoon; **Cover Designer:** Jack Davis; **Illustrator:** M.R. Greenberg; **Printer:** Braun-Brumfield

Printed in the United States of America   10 9 8 7 6 5 4 3 2 1

Human Kinetics
Web site: http://www.humankinetics.com/

United States: Human Kinetics, P.O. Box 5076, Champaign, IL 61825-5076
1-800-747-4457
e-mail: human@hkusa.com

Canada: Human Kinetics, Box 24040, Windsor, ON N8Y 4Y9
1-800-465-7301 (in Canada only)
e-mail: humank@hkcanada.com

Europe: Human Kinetics, P.O. Box IW14, Leeds LS16 6TR, United Kingdom
(44) 1132 781708
e-mail: humank@hkeurope.com

Australia: Human Kinetics, 57A Price Avenue, Lower Mitcham, South Australia 5062
(088) 277 1555
e-mail: humank@hkaustralia.com

New Zealand: Human Kinetics, P.O. Box 105-231, Auckland 1
(09) 523 3462
e-mail: humank@hknewz.com

Here's to the unsung heroes. There are millions of unsung heroes in America, men and women working hard to put bread on the table, pay the bills, clothe their children, hoping today is a little better than yesterday. They may not have the best-looking houses on the block or the newest cars or be able to take a tropical vacation. Their lives are not easy, as they must earn everything they have. Aside from their daily struggles, they show a remarkable capacity to *care* . . . about life, their children, their communities, and their work. They dream of making this a better world, a better place to live and work because of their brains, sweat, and talents. These people are the true superstars!

This book is also dedicated to my loves, Zachary and Katie, and to Elaine Coleman, former Operations and Wellness Manager at The Robert E. Mason Company in Charlotte, North Carolina. For nearly a decade, I had the privilege and pleasure of working with Elaine before her death in 1997 of breast cancer.

CONTENTS

PREFACE

You and I are one among many,
but still we are one.
We cannot do everything,
But still we can do <u>something.</u>

That's what this book is about: doing *something* to enhance the quality of life for millions of Americans who spend one-fourth of their lives at the worksite. Worksite health promotion (WHP) is now recognized as a viable, cost-effective method to combat many of the ailments and stressors that are to blame for poor health and inefficient production at the workplace. In the new millenium we expect to see more and more companies implement the strategies described in this text.

Written primarily for undergraduate and graduate students planning careers in the field of WHP and for those who plan, implement, and direct WHP programs for their companies, this book contains ten chapters divided into four parts, each dealing with an important area of WHP. Part I, Introduction to Worksite Health Promotion, presents an overview of the economic forces affecting America's worksites and how employers are responding to these challenges. Chapter 1 defines and explains WHP and summarizes its history. Arguments for and against the concept of WHP are scrutinized. The case for WHP, evaluated in the light of its influence on overall health and work productivity, is seen to be very strong indeed.

Part II contains four chapters detailing how to get WHP programs up and running at your worksite. Chapter 2 covers the identification and assessment phases of the process and includes a planning framework that illustrates the entire process in a nutshell—from the first stages of identifying key areas to focus WHP programs on, to the final stages of evaluating and restructuring the programs for better success. Chapter 3 explains how to plan WHP programs, including setting appropriate goals, dealing with funding and budgeting concerns, and proposing WHP plans to management. Chapter 4, on implementing WHP programs, discusses marketing issues and suggests specific ways to promote the programs so that they catch on and are popular with the workforce. Chapter 5 explains the necessary stage of program evaluation and how to build evaluation into the program itself.

In the three chapters of part III, readers learn how to build a healthy work environment, where WHP is an accepted and integral part of keeping employees happy and productive while efficiency is improved at the worksite. Chapter 6 focuses on helping a workforce develop a health-minded culture, where health concerns are primary considerations in lifestyle choices. Chapter 7 contains information on the many healthy lifestyle programs and resources available to those who run WHP, including programs on physical fitness, back health, nutrition, prenatal health, smoking-cessation, AIDs, and medical self-care. Chapter 8 presents eleven model WHP programs from across the United States. These programs offer proof of how successful WHP programs can be when planned and run well and can be used as models for starting programs at worksites where WHP has not yet caught on.

Part IV contains two chapters on other considerations in WHP. Many companies have workforces spread over several worksites, which can present problems for WHP that single-site companies don't have. Other companies consider themselves too small for WHP to be an attractive option. Chapter 9 includes information on how to customize WHP programs for small and multisite businesses. Chapter 10, written mainly for the student, presents practical information on how to equip and prepare for a career in the broad field of WHP. The chapter offers tips on how to acquire necessary skills as well as suggestions for landing an internship and preparing to interview with prospective employers.

Considering the growing potential of WHP efforts to enhance American lives and businesses, I hope this book will enhance your personal and professional efforts in the dynamic, ever-changing field of worksite health promotion.

ACKNOWLEDGMENTS

In the 6 years since I wrote my last book on worksite health promotion, many worksites have generously shared information with me in hopes that others could benefit from their ideas. Without their input, this latest text would be less comprehensive. Thanks to those of you who shared. Thanks also to the many students in East Carolina University's worksite health promotion program who made valuable contributions to the book by sharing ideas and editing early drafts of the manuscript.

INTRODUCTION TO WORKSITE HEALTH PROMOTION

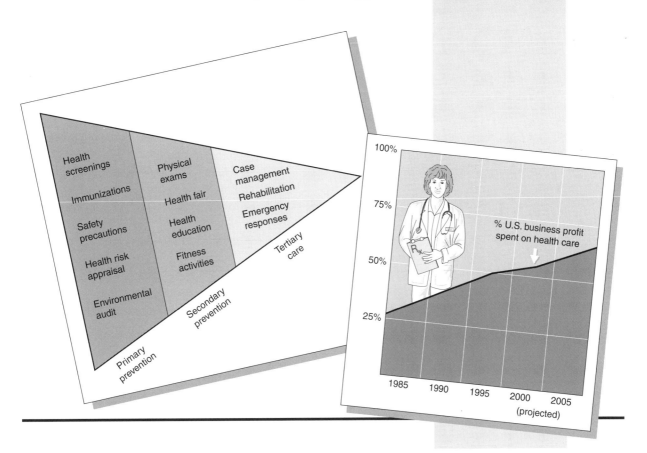

Health
screenings

Immunizations

Safety
precautions

Health risk
appraisal

Environmental
audit

Physical
exams

Health fair

Health
education

Fitness
activities

Case
management

Rehabilitation

Emergency
responses

Tertiary
care

Secondary
prevention

Primary
prevention

100%

75%

50%

25%

% U.S. business profit
spent on health care

1985   1990   1995   2000   2005
(projected)

I

THE CASE FOR WORKSITE HEALTH PROMOTION

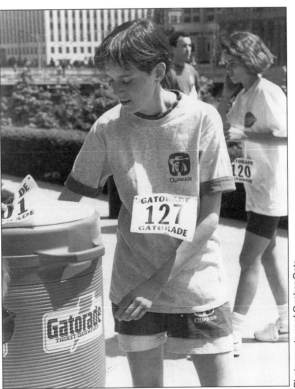

Photo courtesy of Quaker Oats

What is the future of American business? A day rarely passes without our hearing of another lay-off, labor strike, corporate takeover, bankruptcy, or lost lease. These looming possibilities have always been reason for concern in business, but today there is an even greater worry among owners and managers of companies large and small:

the rising cost of paying for employees' health care. Business' portion of America's total health care bill has increased from 18 percent in 1965 to more than 30 percent in 1997. Over 50 percent of business profits are spent annually on employees' and dependents' health care (see figure 1.1).

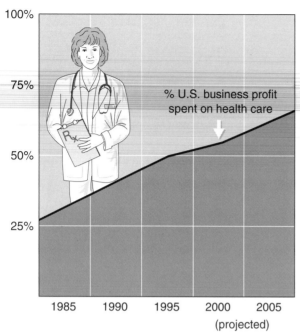

Figure 1.1   Business spending for health care services as an approximate percentage of corporate operating profits.

Although health care cost inflation has slowed in the past decade, it continues to rise nearly twice as fast as general inflation. If this trend continues, within a few years health care spending will consume nearly 20 percent of the nation's **Gross Domestic Product** (or GDP—the total dollar value of all goods and services produced annually by businesses and industries in the United States). This compares to 12 percent in 1990 (see figure 1.2). The combination of rising costs and the rising percentage of those costs borne by business makes health promotion a promising opportunity for American companies.

DEFINING WORKSITE HEALTH PROMOTION

What does the term **health promotion** mean to you? In 1990 the Joint Committee on Health Education Terminology chose to combine health promotion

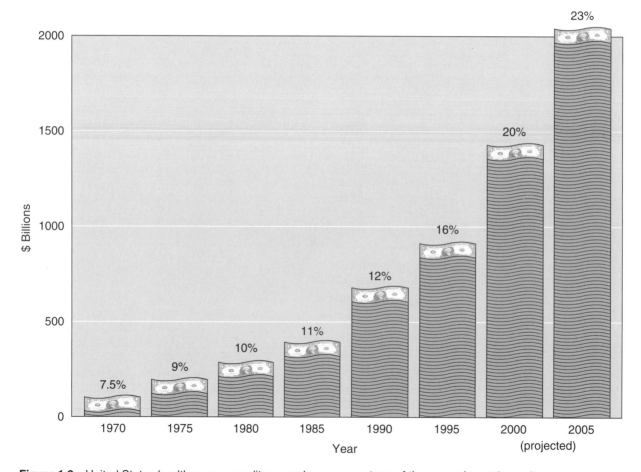

Figure 1.2   United States health care expenditures and as a percentage of the gross domestic product.

and disease prevention and defined this blend as "the aggregate of all purposeful activities designed to improve personal and public health through a combination of strategies, including the competent implementation of behavior change strategies, health education, health protection measures, risk factor detection, health enhancement and health maintenance."

Accordingly, **worksite health promotion** (WHP) is best understood as the combination of educational, organizational, and environmental activities and programs designed to motivate and support healthy lifestyles among a company's employees and their families. The three chief goals of WHP programs are to (1) assess health risks, (2) reduce those health risk factors that can be reduced, and (3) promote socially and environmentally healthy lifestyles.

A Brief History of Worksite Health Promotion

It makes sense that WHP as defined above would help companies contain health expenditures on their employees. Many American businesses have long held that assumption. One of the first worksite-based recreation and fitness programs evolved over a century ago in 1879, when the Pullman Company formed such a program within its own athletic association. Five years later, John R. Patterson, president of National Cash Register, regularly assembled his employees at dawn for pre-work horseback rides. In 1894 he instituted morning and afternoon exercise breaks and, a decade later, built an employee gym. Presumably Patterson was satisfied with the results of these ventures, as in 1911 he added a 325-acre recreation park for his employees.

The growth of worksite recreation and fitness programs leveled off for several decades until the National Employee Services and Recreation Association (NESRA) was formed in 1941 and spearheaded greater interest in employee health. PepsiCo established its physical fitness program in the late 1950s, with American Can and NASA following suit in 1968. Since 1960, Rockwell International has encouraged daily exercise for employees and de-

pendents, while Xerox Corporation has stressed physical fitness since 1965. In the late 1970s, Kimberly-Clark Corporation and Sentry Insurance built state-of-the-art fitness facilities, which served as a major impetus for other companies to follow suit throughout the 1980s. Today NESRA estimates there are over 50,000 organizations with on-site physical fitness programs in the United States and nearly 1,000 employing full-time program directors. Many companies also offer programs for stress management, low back care, smoking cessation, nutrition, and weight control. More than 10,000 U.S. companies have **Employee Assistance Programs** to help employees and dependents with personal problems ranging from substance abuse to emotional stress. Currently over half of all midsize and large American companies offer at least one type of WHP activity, with a growing number of smaller employers catching on. Objective 8.6 of a government document called *Healthy People 2000* challenged more companies to provide WHP programs. As one of the U.S. government's goals to achieve before the year 2000, the objective reads, "…increase to at least 85 percent the proportion of workplaces with 50 or more employees that offer health promotion activities for their employees, preferably as part of a comprehensive employee health promotion program." As of this writing in 1998, the percentage of companies with *comprehensive* WHP programs is about 55 percent, well short of the 85 percent goal for 2000.

In 1992, the U.S. Department of Health and Human Services (HHS) conducted a national survey involving a random sample of 1,507 private sector worksites with 50 or more employees. The worksites were stratified by number of employees and type of industry and had an overall response rate of 74 percent. The key findings of this survey indicate that

- nearly 81 percent of all responding companies offered one or more worksite activities (compared to 66 percent in 1985);
- larger employers, especially those with over 750 employees, are far more likely to have worksite programs than smaller firms;
- WHP activities vary greatly by type of industry; and
- WHP activities vary little across regions.

Why Businesses Offer Worksite Health Promotion

More and more companies are finding that treating employees with respect and care is not only the right thing to do—it's also good business. Why? This question can best be answered by looking at the most common reasons companies give for providing WHP programs:

- **Absenteeism**. Half of all unscheduled absences are due to minor ailments. To battle these ailments, companies offer medical self-care programs to employees and dependents.

- **Accessibility**. The workplace is usually a convenient setting for offering educational and motivational programs to many people at once.

- **Aging workforce**. As American workers age and experience more health problems, many employers are implementing age-appropriate interventions to slow the effects of aging and detect problems earlier.

- **Business contacts**. Health promotion events such as community health fairs and corporate challenge races create new business contacts.

- **Competition**. Concern about retaining employees is prompting companies to provide health club subsidies and other perks to improve morale and increase retention.

- **Health insurance premiums**. Employer-paid health insurance premiums for employees and dependents have risen nearly 1,000 percent since 1960. This statistic alone is enough to move many companies to action. More and more employers are finding WHP to be the best option for combating the huge costs of insurance premiums.

- **Image**. Many corporate leaders realize that successful WHP programs boost a company's image among workers, community, and industry peers.

- **Keeping up with growing national interest**. Nationwide interest in personal health enhancement is reflected in today's print and electronic media coverage. Companies that want to be perceived as innovative pacesetters can't afford to ignore such trends.

- **Productivity**. Since healthy employees generally outperform unhealthy employees, more companies are offering health promotion programs to increase overall productivity.

- **Workers' compensation costs**. Customized WHP programs are successful in many case-management and return-to-work efforts.

Despite all the reasons companies give for offering WHP programs, some people and groups are skeptical about just how valuable even the best WHP program can be in the face of the seemingly insurmountable expense many companies incur because of rising health care costs. In the section that follows we'll look at some of the factors skeptics cite when they argue that WHP programs are not the solution to the problem of skyrocketing health care costs. Later in the chapter, and in subsequent chapters, we'll describe and defend the position that WHP, despite its potential shortcomings, may be the most viable current option for diminishing most of the factors contributing to the escalating costs of health care.

Major Factors Affecting Rising Health Care Costs

Many of those who believe that WHP is not effective in containing business' health care expenses point to factors that contribute to rising health care costs that have little or nothing to do with employee health issues influenced at the worksite. These factors include economic factors, demographic shifts, and chronic health conditions that cannot be eased through typical worksite health programs.

Economic Factors

As is true with any product or service on the market, health care costs fluctuate depending on such factors as inflation, overhead, and operating expenses. When the service is providing medical or health care, some of the expenses necessary for continued operation (e.g., insurance or cost of materials) are much greater than they are for other services, and of course that expense is passed on at least in part to the consumer. If a company offers to its employees the benefit of health insurance, it is the company rather than the individual that takes on all or part of the financial burden passed on by the providing health care agency when the agency's costs escalate. Many companies that absorb this ever-increasing expense must look for ways to cut the costs if they are going to remain in operation. Consequently, companies are becoming more and more interested in the *causes* of rising health care costs as they seek possible ways to manipulate the causes in order to contain costs.

INFLATION

As you would expect, general inflation is a driving force behind rising consumer health care costs. In the Consumer Price Index (a measure of inflation based on the price of a group of commonly purchased goods and services), medical care services often rise twice as fast as other items in the index. This means, for instance, that if the cost of groceries rises 2 percent over 12 months, the cost of health care will rise 2 percent over 6 months. If general inflation continues at the same rate, over the 12 months during which the price of groceries inflates by 2 percent, the price of health care will inflate by 4 percent.

TECHNOLOGICAL GAINS

High-tech equipment is extremely expensive. For example, 20 years ago hospitals used x-rays to view organs and bones; today they use magnetic resonance imagery. But an MRI costs much more than an x-ray, and the consumer must pay the majority of the additional expense. As technological advances occur more rapidly, medical institutions must purchase more and more equipment just to provide what is currently considered standard treatment. If a piece of equipment purchased at great expense in 1999 is improved on in 2002, the institution must purchase the improved piece even before it is finished paying for the piece it will not use anymore. And this is just for standard treatment—what we expect every medical institution to provide. Equipment on the technological cutting-edge costs even more, and the institutions that purchase such equipment must pass

on some of this expense to patients and their insurance companies.

Great strides in technology yield not only improved equipment but also longer lives for many hospitalized patients. Today many illnesses can be diagnosed but not cured; although maintenance programs and life-support systems can keep patients alive for long periods, these interventions carry a huge price tag. Again, this increased expense is paid by insurance companies who in turn pass it on to employers via big increases in the cost of premiums.

CATASTROPHIES, COST-SHIFTING, AND MALPRACTICE INSURANCE

Chronic health conditions, such as being HIV positive, and catastrophic medical cases involving such procedures as transplants or brain surgery, add up to incredibly high medical expenses, some of which are passed on to the patients' employers. Cost-shifting, the "hidden tax" that doctors and hospitals shift to paying customers to compensate for patients who cannot or do not pay their bills, adds one fourth to one third more cost to the average health care bill. Again, much of this expense is taken on by employers. Similarly, the high cost of malpractice insurance for doctors and hospitals is also passed on to paying patients and their employers. A related expense is that more doctors and hospitals now practice "defensive" medicine—doing more procedures than necessary, for example—in an effort to protect themselves from potential lawsuits. The cost of these procedures, necessary or not, partially rest with employers.

DEMOGRAPHIC SHIFTS

Three relatively recent changes in the make-up of the U.S. workforce have significantly influenced health care concerns. These changes, which affect not only physical health but mental health costs as well, are

- the aging of the workforce,
- the overwhelming entry of women into the workplace, and
- the rising proportion of non-Caucasians in the United States.

One of the most significant factors shaping the United States is the aging of Americans. As

Americans live longer, and thus use more health care services, the overall volume of health care services will continue to grow. Middle-age (35- to 54-year-old) workers will make up more than 50 percent of America's workforce by the year 2000. In contrast, younger entry-level workers—especially in the 16- to 34-year-old age group—will soon comprise less than one third of the workforce.

Elder care is one of the fastest-growing needs of many American workers. Currently out of some 30 million adult Americans over 65 years old, about 7.5 million need long-term care. Of those, 1.5 million are in nursing homes. The remaining 6 million receive home care, either within or outside of the health care system. Yet fewer than one half of all companies surveyed expect to provide employees with elder care assistance within the next few years.

Although many older workers can outperform their younger co-workers through greater efficiency, as a group they still encounter greater scrutiny and discrimination from managers and younger workers who often do not understand the aging process and do not appreciate that older workers can be productive in their later years. Some older employees may perceive such treatment as disrespectful and harbor personal and work-related attitude problems that may influence their performance.

Since 1980 the Latin-American population has grown nearly 50 percent while the African-American population has grown almost 20 percent, greatly outpacing the 10-percent growth of Caucasians. This trend has resulted in more non-Caucasians in the workforce, a disproportionate number of whom work in the fast-growing but low-paying service sector of the economy that often provides limited health insurance benefits to employees. Poorly insured workers often delay seeking health care treatment for minor ailments that can worsen and require more expensive health care in the long run. Women are also entering the American workforce at an unprecedented rate. It is estimated that within a few years 60 percent of the labor force will be female. Undoubtedly, these shifts are creating greater stress on working men and women to successfully support their families and balance family life with worklife. The effects of this sort of stress on employees' mental health is a factor that has only recently been taken seriously by many employers.

A 1997 survey of large employers done by the consulting company William M. Mercer suggests that a growing number of organizations are planning to develop programs and policies to help employees with child care, parental leave, elder care, and other emotional and family issues faced by the new workforce. While reviewing the table below, note that in 1993 the Family and Medical Leave Act was passed, requiring companies of 50 or more employees to provide parental leave benefits to all employees, male or female. For companies of fewer than 50 employees, this policy is not required.

Percentage of Employers Offering Service

Service	1997	2005 (projected)
Parental leave	100	100
Flexible scheduling	94	96
Paid time off	93	95
Child care benefits	82	85
Employee assistance	82	85
Multicultural counseling	72	75
Stress management training	52	54
Pre-retirement planning	47	50
Fitness/nutritional counseling	46	50
Elder care	36	43
In-house child care	25	40
Company-funded day care	20	47

CHRONIC HEALTH CONDITIONS

Some employees with chronic health problems such as lupus or diabetes mellitus may not be able to participate in all types of worksite health promotion programs. These chronic conditions, while very expensive to a company, are not the kind of health issues usually targeted by WHP precisely because they are chronic. This is not to say, however, that WHP might not improve the condition as well as the quality of the person's life. It's probably true that WHP can help everyone in some way, regardless of current health status, but some employees with severe health problems will require regular and expensive medical treatment no matter what kind of program they are on.

WHP'S IMPACT ON HEALTH CARE COST FACTORS

The three areas discussed above—economic factors, demographic shifts, and chronic health conditions—are the ones usually cited by skeptics of WHP who believe that a WHP program cannot sufficiently address some of the most significant contributing factors to rising health care costs. While it's true that these areas cannot be directly affected by WHP (e.g., a person with diabetes or anemia cannot overcome his or her affliction by participating in a WHP nutrition program), there are indirect influences of WHP upon these areas with significant positive implications. For instance, while WHP cannot make a person younger and thereby bypass the increased health care expenses associated with age, a good WHP program *can* help older people stay healthy longer and thus avoid dependency on some of the expensive treatments ultimately paid for by the employer. Another example is that although WHP cannot curtail the rising costs of medical care, WHP *can* help more employees avoid the need of this high-priced care—which saves the company money even as medical costs continue to rise. We will revisit discussion of economic variables, demographic shifts, and chronic health conditions in the following chapters. For now it's enough to state our position as being that WHP is a viable option for employers who want to have a healthier workforce and contain medical costs. Inherent shortcomings in what WHP can achieve hardly indicates that a given WHP program is less than entirely worthwhile.

Now that we have discussed some of the health care cost–increasing factors that WHP cannot directly address, let's turn our attention to the most common health risks and costs existing in the workplace. These costs can be directly affected through employee participation in a good WHP program.

HEALTH RISKS AND COSTS

Although we live a little longer than we did in the late 1980s, the health status of the average American in the late 1990s has not improved during the past decade. In fact, we are worse off than we were a decade ago. More women are smoking than ever before and thus risking lung cancer, heart disease, and other smoking-related ailments. And despite the plethora of fat-free foods and exercise options in today's marketplace, more American adults are obese now than ever before.

THE MOST COMMON HEALTH RISKS

Unfortunately, American society's health habits are reflected at most worksites. For example, a 1997 survey of over 400 business owners nationwide suggests that every business has many employees with health problems. Here are the top ten risks indicated in the survey, ranked in order of frequency:

1. Excess stress
2. High blood pressure
3. Cigarette smoking
4. Back injuries
5. Overweight
6. Alcohol abuse
7. High blood cholesterol
8. Drug abuse
9. Depression, and
10. Mental health problems

Independent studies conducted at Steelcase Corporation, Ceridian Corporation (formerly Control Data Corporation), Du Pont Company, Chrysler Corporation, General Motors, and several other companies indicate that most of these identified risk factors are due, in varying degrees, to lifestyle choices. It is these choices, among other concerns, that WHP targets in order to help employees make wiser and healthier decisions about their lifestyles. In the face of all the knowledge they acquire about health, would smokers continue to smoke, drinkers to drink, and procrastinators to procrastinate beginning a fitness program? Yes, evidence strongly indicates that some individuals will maintain their lifestyle almost no matter what and for as long as they are able. However, equally strong evidence indicates that many individuals will in fact change their behavior once they truly understand that it is reducing both the quality and quantity of their life.

COST SHARING

The time is coming—some say it is here—when the availability and cost of specific health care benefits will depend on an employee's lifestyle and risk level. Simply put, lifestyle-related claims such as smoking-induced lung diseases and alcohol-induced motor vehicle accidents—claims directly tied to a person's choice—may not be covered by company-paid insurance. Consequently, health promotion programs may no longer be offered primarily as an employee benefit but as an economic necessity—for the primary purpose of helping high-risk and unhealthy employees reduce their risk factors in order to qualify for health insurance.

In a nationwide poll of 1,500 chief executive officers, 90 percent of the respondents ranked rising health insurance premium costs as their greatest cost concern. When asked how they would contain future health care costs, respondents overwhelmingly (80 percent) said cost-sharing was the preferred method. In fact, over half of the respondents felt cost-sharing was effective in helping control health care expenses. Many employers feel that a moderate cost-sharing arrangement ($250 deductible and 10 percent copayment, for example) can produce substantial cost-savings without discouraging necessary medical care. Some health care economists contend that cost-sharing does very little, if anything, to reduce health care inflation because it merely shifts the cost from employers to employees. In reality, they argue, cost-sharing causes some people to delay seeking treatment when they really

need it. Such delays could lead to needless suffering, gradually worsening health problems, and even higher long-term health care costs. Though these arguments sound reasonable, there is no conclusive evidence that the average cost-sharing arrangement ($350 family deductible and a 15 percent copayment) causes individuals who really need health care to postpone treatment.

HEALTH COSTS AND HEALTH PROMOTION

Considering the high percentage of unhealthy American workers, what can employers expect from their health promotion efforts? Independent studies conducted on employees at Steelcase, Ceridian, Du Pont, General Electric, General Motors, and Chrysler indicate that more than 50 percent of corporate health care costs are due to potentially modifiable (lifestyle) risk factors, such as poor diet, tobacco use, physical inactivity, and the like; as the number of a person's risk factors increases, so does his or her healthcare costs (see figure 1.3); and those

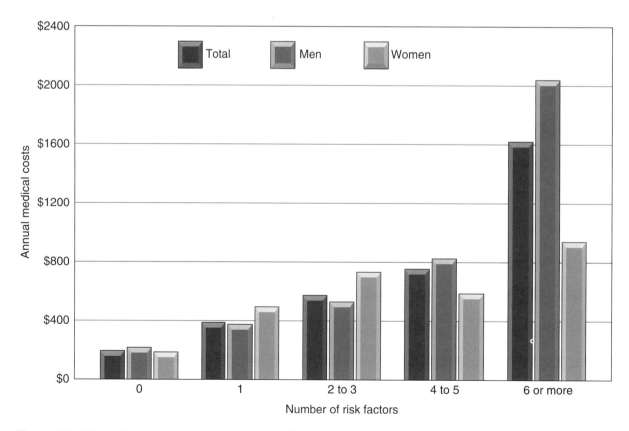

Figure 1.3 The relationship between the number of risk factors and average annual health costs.

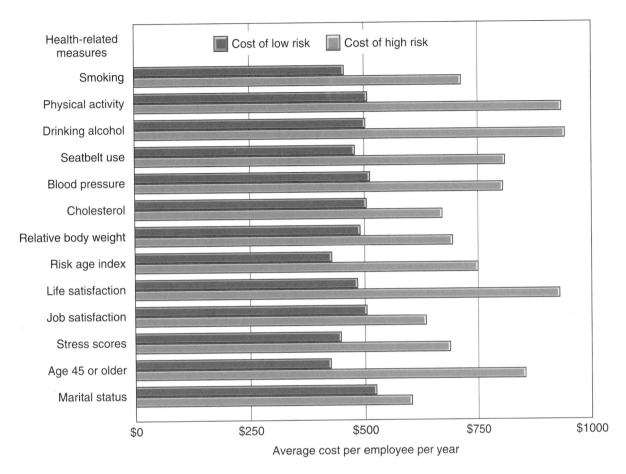

Figure 1.4 Comparisons of medical claims costs according to health risk levels.

people with high-risk lifestyles have higher health care costs than persons with low-risk lifestyles (see figure 1.4).

In particular, a study of 6,000 Chrysler Corporation employees over a period of 3 years showed a strong relationship between an individual's risk level and health care usage. Ten health risks were studied including smoking, body weight, exercise, alcohol use, driving habits, eating habits, stress, mental health, cholesterol level, and blood pressure. Among the key findings were that smokers had 31 percent higher annual claim costs than nonsmokers had; individuals with an elevated risk for obesity had hospital bills 143 percent higher than their low-risk peers; and that of the health behaviors studied, eating habits resulted in the largest difference—41 percent—in costs by risk level between those with poor versus good habits.

Despite its impressive statistics, health promotion is only one piece of the puzzle in building a comprehensive health management framework to create a healthier and more productive workforce

(see figure 1.5). A company's ability to reach this goal depends largely on whether it can consistently do all of the following:

- Provide appropriate health care benefits to employees and their dependents.

- Influence employees and dependents to use health care services regularly and responsibly.

- Encourage employees and dependents to use only quality-oriented, cost-conscious health care providers.

- Monitor and regularly analyze its health care claims data.

Projections for the 21st century suggest that the goals and strategies of WHP will command greater respect from many employers and motivate them to enhance their employee health promotion efforts at the worksite. To reach the desirable goals of improved health in the workplace and health care cost containment, health promotion efforts must appeal to and reach as many employees as possible via both

WORKSITE HEALTH PROMOTION PROGRAMS

Upon mounting evidence that worksite health promotion cuts costs and produces a healthier workforce, more employers are giving WHP programs greater attention. Much of this newfound respect is probably due to the impressive savings reported by 12 companies in *Fortune* magazine. Here are some highlights:

Aetna: Five state-of-the-art centers kept exercisers' health care costs $282 lower than nonexercisers.

L.L. Bean: Due to a healthy workforce, annual health insurance premiums were one half the national average.

Dow Corporation: On-the-job injury strains dropped 90 percent.

Johnson & Johnson: Health screening saved $13 million a year in absenteeism and health care costs.

Quaker Oats: Because of an integrated health management approach, health insurance premiums were nearly a third less than the national average.

Steelcase: Personal health counselors motivated high-risk employees to reduce major risk factors, generating an estimated $20 million over 10 years.

Union Pacific: Reduced hypertension and smoking saves more than $3 million a year.

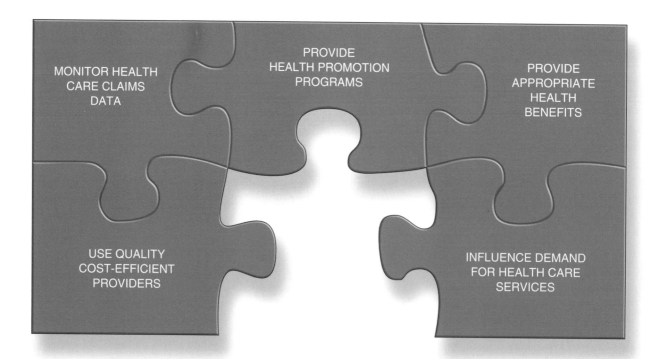

Figure 1.5   Key cost-control strategies that comprise a comprehensive health management framework.

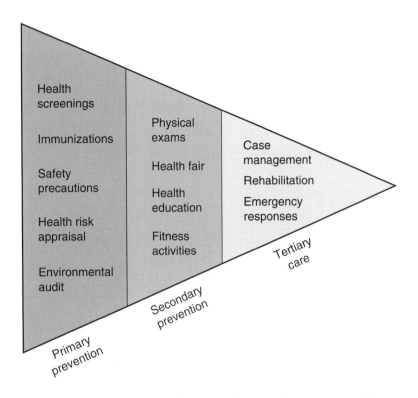

Figure 1.6 Examples of primary prevention, secondary prevention, and tertiary care activities in a worksite setting.

primary and secondary prevention and tertiary care (see figure 1.6).

Of course the odds for developing a healthy workforce and worksite depend on how well employers use their resources in planning appropriate health promotion programs. Chapter 2 introduces a framework to help you focus efforts on building and maintaining an effective WHP program. The chapter also describes basic principles you will want to consider when designing a program.

What Do You Think?

According to a study funded by Marion Merrill Dow, Inc., more employers plan to implement expanded health promotion programs in the next five years. The greatest increases are expected in:

- Employee wellness newsletters
- Weight loss programs
- Lifestyle assessment
- Prostate screenings for men

Do you agree or disagree with these projections? Why? What do you think will be the fastest-growing areas in WHP over the next few years? Which factors will influence this growth?

PLANNING AND IMPLEMENTING WORKSITE HEALTH PROGRAMS

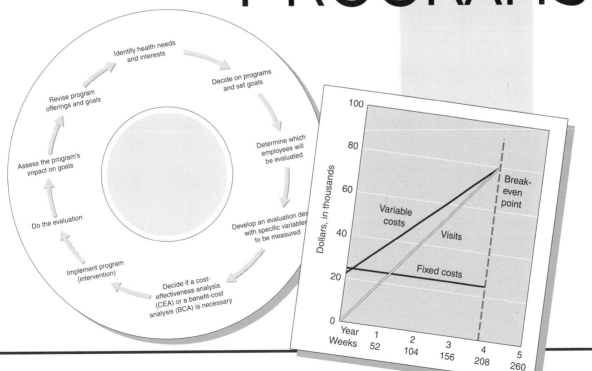

IDENTIFICATION AND ASSESSMENT

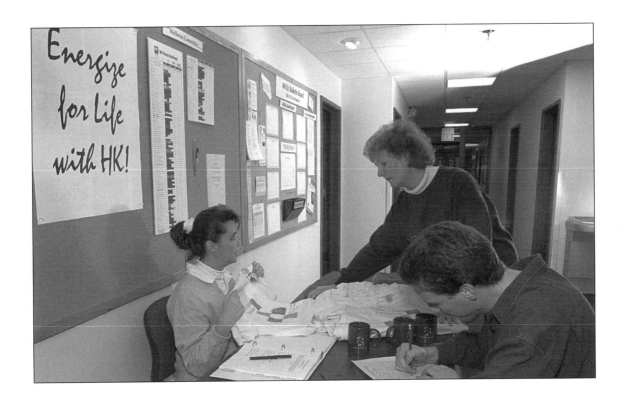

Considering such pressures as downsizing, global competition, and rising production costs, every facet of a business today is under close scrutiny by upper management. As it is a relatively new endeavor for most businesses, worksite health promotion must be planned and positioned even more carefully than other business strategies.

THE PLANNING FRAMEWORK

We have developed a framework to help program planners recognize employee needs and interests prior to planning and implementing appropriate WHP programs. The framework consists of five distinct yet interrelated phases (see figure 2.1):

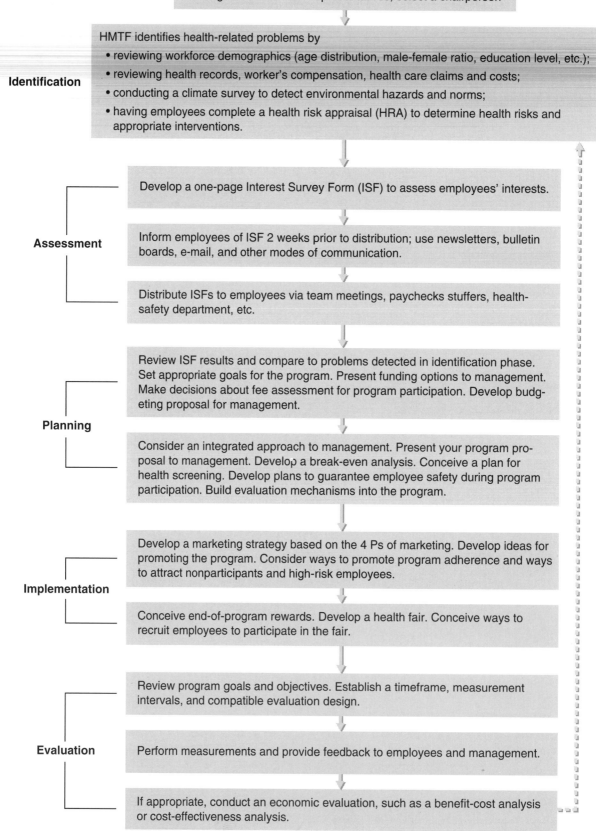

Identification

Form a Health Management Task Force (HMTF) consisting of management and labor representatives; select a chairperson

HMTF identifies health-related problems by

- reviewing workforce demographics (age distribution, male-female ratio, education level, etc.);
- reviewing health records, worker's compensation, health care claims and costs;
- conducting a climate survey to detect environmental hazards and norms;
- having employees complete a health risk appraisal (HRA) to determine health risks and appropriate interventions.

Assessment

Develop a one-page Interest Survey Form (ISF) to assess employees' interests.

Inform employees of ISF 2 weeks prior to distribution; use newsletters, bulletin boards, e-mail, and other modes of communication.

Distribute ISFs to employees via team meetings, paychecks stuffers, health-safety department, etc.

Planning

Review ISF results and compare to problems detected in identification phase. Set appropriate goals for the program. Present funding options to management. Make decisions about fee assessment for program participation. Develop budgeting proposal for management.

Consider an integrated approach to management. Present your program proposal to management. Develop a break-even analysis. Conceive a plan for health screening. Develop plans to guarantee employee safety during program participation. Build evaluation mechanisms into the program.

Implementation

Develop a marketing strategy based on the 4 Ps of marketing. Develop ideas for promoting the program. Consider ways to promote program adherence and ways to attract nonparticipants and high-risk employees.

Conceive end-of-program rewards. Develop a health fair. Conceive ways to recruit employees to participate in the fair.

Evaluation

Review program goals and objectives. Establish a timeframe, measurement intervals, and compatible evaluation design.

Perform measurements and provide feedback to employees and management.

If appropriate, conduct an economic evaluation, such as a benefit-cost analysis or cost-effectiveness analysis.

Figure 2.1 The WHP program planning framework.

1. **Identification**—Identifying health-related problems
2. **Assessment**—Assessing employees interests
3. **Planning**—Locating and applying necessary resources to establish a program
4. **Implementation**—Positioning, promoting, and implementing a program
5. **Evaluation**—Measuring the impact of a program

In this chapter we will deal with the first two phases of the planning framework: Identification and Assessment. Planning, Implementation, and Evaluation will be discussed in chapters 3, 4, and 5, respectively.

Identification deals with the needs of the work force, whereas **assessment** focuses on the desires and intentions of employees and on available resources for approaching problems recognized during identification.

IDENTIFICATION

Identification begins with forming a task force to identify a company's **demographics** (i.e., age distribution, ratio of females to males, education level, and so on); the existing and potential health-related problems of its workforce; and employee interest in participating in programs to improve their health and well-being.

FORMING A TASK FORCE

The fate of a WHP program depends largely on management's philosophy toward employee health issues. When those in management lead healthy lifestyles themselves, they are more inclined to support health enhancement activities at the worksite. This inclination also depends on whether they see strong employee interest in the activities. A very effective way to spark employee interest is to involve workers in planning and implementing the program. Such involvement gives employees a sense of ownership of the program and greatly increases the chances that they'll commit to it.

Although at small worksites the site manager or a supervisor might personally solicit input on employee needs and interests, this personalized approach is not practical for larger organizations. For larger businesses the first step in planning a successful WHP program is to form a **Health Management Task Force** (HMTF) with representatives from both management and employees. HMTF representatives solicit input from all levels of management and labor to ensure that all needs and interests are fully addressed.

The task force should include representatives from every department or category of worker in the company. If a company has union employees, it's important to include union representatives as well. Although the percentage of union workers has dropped annually through the 1990s, about one of every seven American workers still belongs to a union. Unions remain a dynamic force in many worksites and can enhance WHP efforts by encouraging employee participation and working closely with management.

In all worksite settings, the HMTF needs a leader. This person should be respected by employees and managers, skilled in working with small and large groups, sincerely interested in employee health issues, and able to be objective so that the task force is fair to all parties. Other key issues to consider when organizing an HMTF include the following:

- Source of main leadership (from management or employee ranks)
- Number of management and nonmanagement members
- Meeting schedule (weekly or monthly)
- Who will receive the HMTF reports
- Primary role of the HMTF (e.g., planning, implementing, etc.)
- Power or influence of the HMTF (e.g., advisory only)
- Compensation (e.g., release time from job, t-shirts for members)

Once a task force and its leader have been selected, the next steps are to identify health-related problems at the worksite and to evaluate overall interest in programs that WHP might offer.

IDENTIFYING HEALTH-RELATED PROBLEMS

Since employee health needs and interests vary from worksite to worksite, the HMTF should carefully assess each workforce for specific problems. For example, is the number of low back injuries high enough to justify a healthy back program? How big a problem is smoking at the worksite? Does the worksite promote personal health? What days and times are best to offer particular programs? Will employees resist the programs unless they are paid or rewarded in some way? These are just a few questions that the task force should consider.

An early responsibility for the HMTF is to solicit input from workers at all job levels to ensure that employee needs and interests are accurately identified. Identification strategies should include analyzing

- workforce demographic data,
- employee health records,
- health care claims and costs,
- workers' compensation claims and cost data,
- worksite environment, and
- health risk appraisal data.

At the end of the chapter appears a Personal Health Questionnaire you can distribute to employers to gather more information during the identification phase (see pp. 29-32).

WORKFORCE DEMOGRAPHIC DATA

The minimum **demographic data** the task force should acquire for the worksite include the ratios of male employees to female employees, salaried employees to hourly employees, and day workers to night workers; age groups; ethnicity; and the percentage of workers with dependents. This information will be key in planning what kinds of programs will be most useful and appropriate for WHP.

EMPLOYEE HEALTH RECORDS

Because of the need to protect each employee's medical privacy and health status, these data should be accessed and reviewed only by authorized personnel. In many cases this information can be used to compile a Group Health Data Sheet, listing a worksite's most prevalent health problems. A sample data sheet is shown in table 2.1.

HEALTH CARE CLAIMS AND COST DATA

The availability and specificity of health care claims and cost data vary greatly from worksite to worksite.

The data may be handled by a specific department or, in other cases, an employer may need to ask its insurer or third-party administrator to provide these data. Tables 2.2 and 2.3 show claims and costs by **major diagnostic category** (MDC) and subcategories that are identified by a four-digit **International Classification of Disease** (ICD) code. At a minimum, claims data should provide the following:

- Major diagnostic category and preferably ICDs
- Number of claims and charges per MDC
- Inpatient versus outpatient claims and charges per MDC
- Employee-specific versus dependent-specific claims and charges per MDC

These data will help the task force recognize which WHP programs might be most beneficial and estimate potential savings for the company if a successful WHP is implemented.

WORKERS' COMPENSATION CLAIMS DATA

These data, typically handled by the health and safety, risk management, or human resources department, show the incidence and types of injuries resulting in work-related absence and/or disability, and any employer-paid compensation paid to injured employees. Like health care claims and costs data, this information helps the task force target programs and is useful in calculating possible savings if a successful WHP program is established at a company.

Table 2.1 A Sample Data Sheet		
	Data sheet (workforce of 200 employees)	
Health condition	**Number**	**Percentage**
Low back injury	47	23.5
Cigarette smoker	42	21.0
Overweight or obese	40	20.0
High blood pressure	28	14.0
Joint injury	18	9.0
Chronic bronchitis	17	8.5
High blood cholesterol	15	7.5
Hearing loss in one ear	10	5.0

Table 2.2	A Sample Listing of Major Diagnostic Category (MDCs)		
MDC	Number of claims	Total charges	Charge per claim
1. Infectious	2	$ 948	$ 474
2. Neoplasm	5	58,924	11,784
3. Endo/nutr.	4	1,880	470
4. Blood	0	0	0
5a. Mental	10	8,900	890
5b. Alcohol/drug	7	5,180	740
6. Nervous	2	1,960	980
7. Circulatory	3	13,500	4,500
8. Respiratory	3	1,050	350
9. Digestive	4	1,808	452
10. Genitourinary	17	6,613	389
11a. Pregnancy	2	6,440	3,230
11b. Newborn	2	2,220	1,110
11c. Perinatal	1	1,890	1,890
12. Skin	7	1,575	225
13. Muscoskeletal	14	7,840	560
14. Congenital	0	0	0
15. S/S/Ill-defined	47	3,150	225
16. Acc/Inj/Poisoning	4	1,504	376
17. Other, ill-defined	8	3,192	399

CLIMATE OBSERVATION

At many worksites employees are randomly monitored for the effects of certain risk factors and work styles on their health status. Depending on the nature of their work and their personal habits, some employees are more likely than others to experience certain problems. Ailments commonly associated with particular risk factors are shown in the adjacent table.

Environmental Checksheet

An Environmental Checksheet can be used to identify existing and potential problems at a worksite, especially those due to working patterns or environmental factors, such as the percentage of time workers are doing physical labor. Since each worksite and workforce is unique, the sample checksheet on pages 22-23 can be modified to suit particular needs (see figure 2.2).

Risk factor	Types of problems
Sedentary jobs	Musculoskeletal, circulatory, and mental health ailments
Smoking	Circulatory and respiratory ailments
Unhealthy eating	Fatigue, circulatory and digestive ailments
Substance abuse	Drug dependence, hyperactivity, apathy, absenteeism, accidents
Low water intake	Urinary tract infections
Poor body mechanics	Musculoskeletal ailments

HEALTH RISK APPRAISAL

One of the most common identification tools used at the worksite is a **health risk appraisal** (HRA),

Table 2.3   A Health Care Claim Report Listing of ICD Claims Within Selected Major Diagnostic Categories

	Highest cost MDCs (total charges) with ICDs		
MDC/ICD code	Number of claims	Total charges	Charge per claim
3. *Neoplasm*			
172.0 Skin	2	$ 7,192	$ 3,596
174.4 Breast	1	19,484	19,484
183.0 Ovary	1	15,400	15,400
188.3 Bladder	1	16,848	16,848
5a. *Mental*			
300.0 Anxiety	4	1,927	481
300.4 Depression	5	5,975	1,195
301.3 Explosive personality	1	998	998
7. *Circulatory*			
402.1 Hypertension	1	3,256	3,256
414.0 Atherosclerosis	1	7,777	7,777
455.0 Hemorrhoids	1	2,467	2,467

A Sample Environmental Checksheet

Nature of work—

1. Percentage of workers doing physical labor ____%

2. Percentage sitting most of time ____%

3. Percentage of workers standing ____% sitting ____% lifting ____%

Behaviors—

1. Percentage of workers operating video display terminals (VDTs) ____%;

   Are VDT stations equipped with filtered screens? ____

   Wrist and hand rests? ____

   Indirect lighting? ____

   Positioned appropriately for employee's height, reach, and posture? ____

   If not, what improvements are necessary?

   _____

   _____

2. Percentage of workers walking, standing, or sitting with poor posture ____%

3. Percentage of workers doing a lot of lifting ____%

   Percentage lifting over 10 pounds per lift ____%

4. Percentage of workers smoking on the job ____%

   Smoking in other areas where smoking is permitted ____%

Other significant behaviors (list):

Environmental health and safety hazards—

1. Is the work environment noisy? ____ If so, where? _____

2. Is the work environment hot? ____ cold? ____ If so, where? _____

3. Is the lighting adequate? ____ If not, where? _____

4. Are there fumes, vapors, or mists in the air?____ If so, describe _____

5. Any employees exposed to substances that are toxic or caustic (burning)? ____ If so, describe

   _____

   _____ Are employees properly protected? ____

(continued)

Figure 2.2   A sample environmental checksheet.

6. Any employees around flying objects? _____
   If so, where? _____
   _____ Are employees pro-
   perly protected? ____

7. Any employees likely to injure themselves
   through improper lifting? ____ If so, where?
   _____

8. Any areas that are slick or where employees
   may fall? ____ If so, where? _____
   _____

9. Areas where employeees may be caught in,
   on, or between machinery? ____ If so, where?
   _____

Safety promotion and injury prevention—

1. Are warning notices posted at high-risk areas?
   ____ If not, where are notices needed? _____
   _____

2. Are visible posters displayed to motivate
   safety practices? ____ If not, where are they
   needed? _____
   _____

3. Are safety records posted? ____ If not, where
   should they be posted? _____
   _____

4. Workers in high-risk areas wearing proper clothing, safety gloves, hard hats, goggles, protective
   shoes? ____ If not, where are they needed?
   _____
   _____

Summary

1. Nature of work for most employees is physical
   ____ Mental ____

2. Most significant behaviors displayed among
   workers include

   a. _____

   b. _____

   c. _____

3. Degree of risk associated with health and safety
   hazards

   a. high ____ Why? _____

   b. fair ____ Why? _____

   c. low ____

Investigator's signature

_____

Date _____

Figure 2.2   *(continued)*

which seeks to identify, assess, and reduce risk. This approach to preventive medicine is called **prospective medicine** and is defined as a discipline concerned with the identification of the individual's changing risks of disease and the recognition of his earliest deviations from health. Prospective medicine aims to promote health and prevent disease, extending useful life expectancy by complementing medical care with the reduction of long-term health risks.

In the early 1960s the concept of prospective medicine was expanded to include a comprehensive concern for an individual's total, and changing, spectrum of risks. Throughout the 1960s and 1970s, as research added to the medical understanding of risk, appraisal instruments were developed, refined, and introduced in public health, university, and worksite settings. Currently there are approximately 30 commercialized HRA instruments. Typi-

cally, an HRA will ask employees for information in the following areas:

- Current health status
- Personal and family medical history
- Daily activities and hobbies
- Major life experiences
- Healthy habits
- Safety habits
- Demographic details

This compiled information then assists management or the WHP staff in identifying current risks and possibly reducing the causing factors of health risks.

Despite their widespread appeal, HRAs are not simple to use and have the following potential drawbacks:

- If they are used carelessly HRAs can cause anxiety, depresson, confusion, and needless expenses for medical care.

- Understanding the highly quantitative nature of HRAs often requires an above average educational background.

- An HRA is not designed to replace a physical exam or other screenings performed by a qualified health care provider.

Since HRA instruments vary in many features, it's a good idea to review several formats before selecting one. Here are some questions to consider before purchasing an HRA:

- Does a single fee cover everything for the HRA, or are there separate fees for the questionnaire, processing, and printing of reports?

- What discount is available with a bulk order?

- Does the database reflect a population similar to your workforce?

- What reading level is required to read the HRA?

- Is a Group Report (Summary) included in the standard package?

- What's the turnaround time?

The Society of Prospective Medicine has published *The Handbook of Health Risk Appraisals*, an informative book that highlights features for each HRA. For more information contact the Society of Prospective Medicine at 341 Ridder Road South, Sewickley, PA 15143. Their phone number is 412-749-1177.

SUMMARY

The identification phase of the planning framework is crucial in that it's at this time you will bring together data to base your WHP program upon. You must accumulate enough data during identification to be able to defend or justify your judgments in designing your WHP programs. For example, it's important to collect different information during the assessment phase to illuminate employee interest in and willingness to participate in potential WHP programs.

ASSESSMENT

As the identification process winds down, program planners should move into assessment, the second phase of the planning framework. This stage focuses on the desires and intentions of employees and on ways to deal with problems recognized during the identification phase.

INTEREST SURVEY FORM

A popular assessment tool is an **interest survey form** (ISF). In preparing an ISF, program planners should strive to limit it to one page and consider whether a specific or generic format is most appropriate. For example, a generic format, shown in the box on the next page, is a good way to assess employee interests in a variety of programs and activities. However, some organizations wish to assess interest for a specific program (exercise, for example) and thus choose to limit the ISF to questions about that program.

PUBLICIZING AND DISTRIBUTING THE ISF

To improve the response rate, employees should be informed of the interest survey form at least twice before they are distributed. Modes of communication include

- company newsletter,
- electronic message boards,
- computer e-mail,
- flyers,
- paycheck stuffers, and
- bulletin board displays in key locations.

Within a couple of days of publicizing the ISF, the forms should be distributed either personally to each employee or to his or her mailbox. You might also include a note encouraging all employees to respond, even if their only response is "Not interested."

TELL US WHERE YOU STAND!

Please check the programs you would like to see offered.

____ General health care (ways to become or stay healthy and fit)

____ Walking

____ High blood pressure

____ First aid and CPR

____ Nutrition

____ Aerobic exercise

____ How to quit smoking

____ Weight control

____ Prenatal health

____ Back pain

____ Managing stress

____ Self-care

____ Other (describe):

_____

Please also list your three favorite topics in order of interest:

1. _____   2. _____   3. _____

Would you participate in any of these programs at the worksite on your own time?   Yes ___   No ___

What days would you prefer?   M ___   Tu ___   W ___   Th ___   F ___   Sat ___   Sun ___

What times would you prefer?   Before work ___   During breaks ___   During lunch ___   After work ___

What is the biggest barrier for you to overcome to participating in a worksite program (no time, too lazy, etc.)? _____

Comments: _____

Please return this survey to _____ by _____

Stay tuned for future details!

If by the due date for the form to be returned you have received less than 75 percent of the forms, you might distribute a reminder and then extend the due date by a few days. If you still have less than a 75 percent response rate after the extended due date, you might need to request that supervisors ask their employees personally if they returned the form.

ASSESSING ISF FEEDBACK

Once the ISFs are returned, the program planner will need to compare the feedback on the forms with the employee needs identified earlier in the identification phase. Often the identified needs and expressed interests by the employees will conflict. For example, suppose after the ISF has been returned, the program planner has the following information to work with:

Channel	Feedback
Employee health records	37% of employees have been treated for a degree of low back pain
	40% of employees have ailments due to smoking
Environmental checksheet	Some improper lifting
	Employees indicate eyestrain at the computer
Health risk appraisal	38% of employees have family histories of lung cancer
Health claims summary	Pregnancy is most common
	Musculoskeletal (low back) is most expensive

Information received via the ISF during assessment phase: the top five interests cited by employees

1. Walking
2. Weight control
3. Back pain
4. Prenatal health
5. How to quit smoking

As you can see, the data collected during the identification phase indicates that back injuries and back pain could be a serious concern at your worksite. However, back pain ranks third on collected ISFs. Since the information and feedback gathered during the two phases differ, how should a program planner decide which needs and interests should receive priority? One way is to contact other area worksites; if they offer the specific program you're considering, they can tell you how well it has been received. Second, you can review the professional literature to determine what types of programs have the greatest potential for achieving a particular goal and weigh this information along with employee preferences and identified needs in a feasibility grid.

For example, in considering a low back injury prevention program, a review of the research literature by the program planner revealed that low back injuries occur most frequently in employees with weak abdominal muscles, poor low back flexibility, or improper lifting techniques. Thus, a back health program would have more impact if it were designed to

- appeal to at-risk employees,
- strengthen employees' abdominal muscles,
- enhance employees' low back and hamstring flexibility, and
- motivate individuals to lift properly.

These objectives can then be plugged into a feasibility grid (see table 2.4), representing the steps that must be completed to reach program-specific goals, along with outcome criteria, determined in the identification phase, and employees' preferences expressed in the ISF.

According to the sample comparison shown in table 2.4, low back programs may have the greatest potential for making a positive impact on most of the criteria. Although a worksite may choose to offer a low back program independent of other programs, the grid might suggest that better results may be obtained from integrative programming—that is,

merging other preferences (such as exercise and weight control) with the low back program.

Let's look again at the conflicting data we have received during the identification phase and from the ISF. Data collected at the identification phase clearly show that smoking is a problem that should be addressed at your worksite, but "how to quit smoking" receives relatively low interest on the ISF compared to "walking." What should you do? You might ask experienced WHP program directors and check the available literature to see whether smoking cessation programs or walking programs have had better WHP success rates. If walking has fared well as a WHP program, you might choose to launch health promotion at your worksite with a walking program, because of its proven success elsewhere. As employees begin to experience the health benefits of exercise, you might then implement the idea of smoking cessation as a way of improving one's comfort level while walking, or of removing limitations to walking goals. On the other hand, if you had begun health promotion at your worksite with the smoking cessation program, you might have met with immediate resistance—because this was not the program employees expressed most interest in—and thereby reduced interest in both the walking program and the WHP program overall.

You can see that assessing feedback from the ISF properly involves more than a simple quantitative evaluation. To make the best use of the ISF, you'll need to compare the results with other data and do the follow-up research necessary for viewing the ISF data in the most useful light.

ASSESSING WHAT WILL MOTIVATE EMPLOYEES

Closely related to what interests employees is the issue of what will motivate them to follow up on their expressed interests. A good way to determine incentives is to survey employees via a questionnaire. Publicize an **Incentive Survey** like the sample shown on the bottom of the next page and distribute it along with the ISF. Adapt this sample to your own company based on preliminary projections of your budget, program offerings, and number of employees expected to participate. The survey should give you a general idea of how to attract employees, which you can combine later with the information

Table 2.4   A Sample Feasibility Grid

	Key: **H** = high **M** = moderate **L** = low		
	Program ranking on ISF		
	1st **Exercise walking**	**2nd** **Weight control**	**3rd** **Low back**
CRITERIA (Potential impact of program on specific criteria)			
A. *Process criteria*			
1. Appeal to employees	H	H	M
2. Measurability	M	H	H*
3. Strengthen abdomen	M	L	M
4. Improve back flexibility	L	L	H*
5. Motivate proper lifting	L	L	H*
B. *Outcome criteria*			
1. Reduce the number of on-the-job back injuries	L	L	H*
2. Reduce absenteeism due to low back injuries	L	L	H*
3. Reduce low back–related health care costs	L	L	H*

*Based on findings of 14 independent studies reviewed by the author.

TELL US WHAT YOU WANT!

As you probably know by now, we are planning to launch a new program to promote interest in employee health and well-being. We hope that you will be enthusiastic about the program and want to participate. With that in mind, we're now considering what incentives would be most popular with the majority of employees. If you'll take a few minutes to think about and fill in the short form below, we'll know better how to make our new program more appealing to you. Please indicate your preferences by checking the appropriate blanks below. Thank you!

	Value to you		
Incentive	**High**	**Moderate**	**Low**
T-shirt	_____	_____	_____
Gift certificate from _____ (please fill in the blank)	_____	_____	_____
Trophy/plaque	_____	_____	_____
Wellness day off work	_____	_____	_____
Certificate	_____	_____	_____
Personal health manual	_____	_____	_____
Sweepstakes	_____	_____	_____
Free health appraisal	_____	_____	_____
Health club discount	_____	_____	_____
Exercise clothing	_____	_____	_____
Exercise shoes	_____	_____	_____
Health insurance premium discount	_____	_____	_____
Photo in newsletter	_____	_____	_____
Other (please list):			

on resources that you will gather during the planning phase, discussed in chapter 3.

SUMMARY

Assessment is a crucial phase in the framework for planning your WHP programs. Misjudgments during this phase can have seriously detrimental impact on the WHP program. Accurate assessments, however, can get WHP started off on the right track, greatly increasing the chances for long-term success.

What Would You Do?

Suppose a workforce comprised of 40-percent smokers expressed on the Interest Survey Form an interest in walking and stress management. However, smoking appears to be the most prevalent risk factor in the workforce, and you feel some smokers would like to quit. Some research indicates smokers are more likely to quit if they begin an exercise program and learn to manage stress. You assume that some smokers, though not all, would participate in a walking program. You also assume that many of those who expressed interest in walking and managing stress are among the 60 percent of nonsmokers. What approach would you take in developing your next program to address all of these issues? Describe and justify your strategy.

PERSONAL HEALTH QUESTIONNAIRE

Please complete the following questionnaire and return it to _____.

We will contact you to schedule your first consultation. If you have any questions, please call _____.
All information is confidential!

Name_____ Employee number (if applicable) _____

Sex: M ___ F ___ Birthdate _____ Dept./Title _____

Phone: Home ( ) _____ Work ( ) _____

Emergency contact _____ Phone _____

A. Activity Profile

Intensity and Exertion (please circle one)

	Low		Moderate		High
1. Level of physical activity at work.	1	2	3	4	5
2. Level of physical activity at leisure.	1	2	3	4	5

3. Do you currently exercise regularly?   Yes __ No __

4. Number of times per week.   1–2   3–4   5–6   Over 6

5. How long do you exercise daily (minutes)?   <15   15–30   30–45   >45

6. Briefly describe your exercise program or workout:

_____

_____

If you answered No to #3 above, when was the last time you exercised, and what type of activity did you do? _____

_____

B. Biomedical Profile

1. Name(s) of your physician(s): _____

2. Date of last complete medical exam _____

3. What is your resting blood pressure? _____ Not sure _____

4. What is your resting heart rate? _____ Not sure _____

5. What is your blood cholesterol level? _____ Not sure _____

6. What is your ratio of total cholesterol to HDL cholesterol? _____ Not sure _____

7. What is your body fat percentage? _____ Not sure _____

(continued)

8. Do you have, or have you ever had, any of the following? Check all that apply.

Condition	Past	Present	Condition	Past	Present
Angina	____	____	Extra heartbeats	____	____
Arthritis	____	____	Heart attack	____	____
Asthma	____	____	Heart murmur	____	____
Back pain	____	____	High blood pressure	____	____
Bronchitis	____	____	Leg cramps	____	____
Cancer	____	____	Pneumonia	____	____
Diabetes	____	____	Rheumatic fever	____	____
Dizziness/fainting	____	____	Scarlet fever	____	____
Emphysema	____	____	Stroke	____	____
Epilepsy	____	____	Varicose veins	____	____
Muscle weakness	____	____	Muscle pain	____	____
Bone injuries	____	____	Bone pain	____	____
Surgery*	____	____	Shortness of breath	____	____

*Date of surgery _____ Type of surgery _____

9. Explanation/comments on any of the above: _____
_____

10. Other diseases/injuries/medical problems you have or have had: _____
_____

11. Do you have any medical problem or injury that might make it difficult to exercise?

Yes ____ No ____ If yes, explain _____
_____

C. Family History

Indicate the number of blood relatives (mother, father, siblings) who have had the following conditions:

Condition	No. of relatives	Condition	No. of relatives
Alcoholism or drug addiction	____	High blood pressure	____
Heart attack	____	Stroke	____
Heart attack before age 60	____	Obesity (30% or more above ideal weight)	____
Diabetes	____		

(continued)

D. Health Inventory and Lifestyle

1. Height _____ Weight _____ Weight at age 21 _____

2. What do you consider to be a good weight for you? _____

3. Have you ever been on a diet prescribed by a doctor or registered dietitian? Yes ____ No ____

   How many pounds did you lose? _____ In how many weeks? _____

4. Do you currently smoke tobacco products? No ____ (skip to #8) Yes ____

   ____ cigarettes; packs per day ____

   ____ cigars; number per day ____

   ____ pipe; pouches per day ____

5. How many years have you smoked? _____

6. What is the primary reason you smoke? _____

   _____

7. Have you ever tried quitting? No ____ Yes ____ By what method? _____

8. Do you drink alcoholic beverages? No ____ (skip to #9) Yes ____

   ____ beer; cans per day ____

   ____ wine; glasses per day ____

   ____ liquor; shots per day ____

9. What types of caffeinated beverages do you drink?

   ____ caffeinated coffee; cups per day ____

   ____ tea; cups per day ____

   ____ cola; cans per day ____

10. Place a check mark beside those foods you eat at least once a day:

___ Whole milk	___ Hard cheese	___ Eggs
___ Butter	___ Ice cream	___ Chocolate
___ Deep-fried foods	___ Cake/pie/donuts	___ Cold cuts
___ Sausage/ham/bacon	___ French fries	___ Fast foods
___ Chips		

(continued)

11. How much stress do you have in an average day?

_____ More than the average person

_____ About the same as the average person

_____ Less than the average person

12. How do you manage stress? _____

_____

_____

E. Personal Interests

Check the programs you would like to participate in.

___ Low-impact aerobics	___ Basketball
___ Cycling	___ Bowling
___ Low back health	___ Softball
___ Nutrition	___ Volleyball
___ Weight control	___ Other (list)
___ Weight lifting	
___ Walking	
___ Smoking cessation	
___ Lifestyle management	
___ Parenting	
___ Caring for elders	
___ Self-care	
___ Using health care benefits	
___ Other (list)	

_____

_____

Thank you. Your feedback will help us plan programs and activities to help you achieve your personal health goals.

C H A P T E R

3

PLANNING WORKSITE
HEALTH PROGRAMS

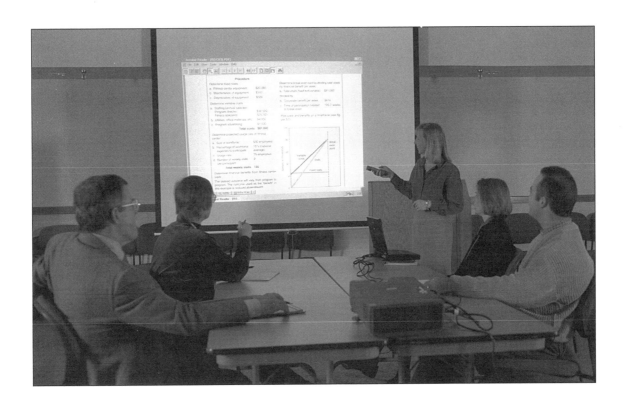

As budgets get tighter and the demands to justify spending become greater, health promotion planners must plan better than ever. In this chapter you will learn more about issues to consider during the planning phase of the framework introduced last chapter (see p. 17). The results of the identification and assessment phases discussed in chapters 2 and 5 should direct programming decisions. For example, as you prepare strategies to deal with the problems identified during phases 1 and 2, you should review the collected data in order to answer three questions about each problem:

1. How prevalent is the problem?

2. What are the consequences and the causes of the problem?

3. Which workers in the company are at greatest risk?

Let's see how this process works by imagining a company that is considering a low back injury prevention program. Program planners in this company begin by asking question number 1: *How prevalent is the problem?* Data gathered during the first phase tell them that nearly one of every four employees reported a low back injury over the past year. These numbers constitute a pervasive problem, so the planners proceed to the next question: *What are the consequences and the causes of the problem?* Reviewing the data, planners discover that a third of those reporting low back pain missed more than 2 weeks of work during the previous year. What's more, they learn that nearly half of the employees with back pain do not always use proper lifting methods. This information indicates to WHP planners that a program should be developed to address low back injuries. Once this decision has been made, the third question is asked: *Which workers in the company are at greatest risk?* Again reviewing data gathered during the identification phase, planners find that the majority of those who reported low back injury or low back pain were men under 45 who worked in the shipping, foundry, or quality control departments.

So, after asking the three questions above, program planners understand that

- there is a need for a low back injury program,

- a consequence of the problem is high absenteeism,

- a cause of the problem is that some workers do not know or do not use proper lifting technique, and

- the program should be targeted mainly at men under 45 who work in one or more of three specific departments.

Armed with this information, the WHP program developers can now proceed through several important steps, including (though not always in this order):

1. Setting appropriate goals for the program

2. Funding and budgeting the program

3. Deciding whether to recommend to management an integrated program (i.e., WHP set within an already established department such as Human Resources) or a program that exists on its own, outside of established departments

4. Presenting to management a proposal to implement the program

5. Screening employees for health risks

6. Incorporating within the program ways to evaluate the program's effectiveness

7. Giving the program a trial run

Each of these steps in the planning process will be discussed in detail in the following sections.

SETTING APPROPRIATE GOALS

For convenience we'll continue to use our example of a company where low back injury has been recognized as a pervasive problem among employees. During this first step of the planning phase, the company's WHP program planners need to establish goals that are realistic enough to attain and yet demanding enough to bring about a clear improvement in the problem area.

Both the research literature and common sense tell us that there is a connection between improper lifting technique and back injury or pain. In our example company, almost half of the employees with back injury or pain do not always use proper lifting technique—thus it's reasonable to assume that reports of back injury and pain could decrease up to 50 percent if all employees lifted properly. If this is the case, would a program outcome of reducing lower back injury reports by 50 percent be a suitable goal? The answer is probably not. Although 50 percent sounds like a high percentage under most circumstances, in this case the percentage should be higher. Considering how relatively simple it should be to reduce by nearly half the number of total low back injuries reported (because a single intervention—proper lifting technique—is sufficient rather than multiple interventions), a good low back program should strive for closer to a 75 percent success rate. This would mean that 25 percent of all back injury reports would need to be addressed through interventions other than training for proper lifting technique. This sounds like a realistic expectation.

Each case must be evaluated individually to establish a suitable goal for each program. For a low back program at this hypothetical company, a 75 percent reduction is demanding yet realistic. Such a high reduction would probably *not* be a realistic goal for a WHP smoking-cessation or nutrition program.

FUNDING WHP PROGRAMS

For most companies the decision whether to try a WHP program comes down to funding. Since one of the biggest challenges for a health promotion program director is to convince management that WHP is a way *to control costs* while improving health and well-being among the work staff, the issue of how much it will cost to initiate a WHP program can be a delicate one.

Unfortunately, in many work settings WHP programs are viewed as the "new kids on the block" and thus must operate with limited funding from management. Sometimes program planners can dodge this situation by positioning their programs in places where they'll receive more visibility and management support. For instance, in many companies WHP programs are housed in human resources, personnel, or health and safety departments. Thus they operate within a departmental budget rather than on a separate budget. A program may or may not do well under such an arrangement. If, for example, the department within which the WHP program is located experiences an unexpected expense, crucial dollars for funding health promotion may no longer exist. This is a risk worth taking in the view of many program directors, especially if one can request a separate budget within the department to ensure adequate resources. In any case, the strategy of receiving greater funding for health programs by integrating them with another department is worth considering. (See Integrated Health Management on p. 38.)

ASSESSING FEES FOR PARTICIPATION IN WHP PROGRAMS

Some employers try to offset part of the expense of WHP by charging employees modest fees for participating in programs and activities. For instance,

we surveyed several companies with on-site fitness centers and found that annual fees for using the center ranged from $80 to over $500 (most charged between $100 and $200). While some worksites contend that fees are financially necessary and actually boost participation rates, other companies choose not to charge employees fees for programs and activities, hoping that free participation and access will be an incentive.

ALTERNATIVE FUNDING SOURCES

General Dynamics in San Diego finances its WHP program with revenue from on-site food and beverage vending sales. In 1949 the company subcontracted the machines through a nationwide food service company and, in return for reporting repair and servicing needs, receives 18 percent of the gross vending sales. This kind of innovative funding is available to many companies with the vision to recognize them. A WHP program planner should explore such funding possibilities with management.

BUDGETING FOR SUCCESS

WHP program planners need to develop a sound proposal to be reviewed by management. This proposal must include itemized costs and clearly indicate how proposed programs and resources can meet company needs. Sample costs for conducting a low back stretching and flexibility program in a worksite of 300 employees are reflected in table 3.1.

Based on the comparison shown in the table, the projected benefit ($86,894) exceeds the projected program costs ($81,576), indicating that a low back program on company time would be a worthy investment.

BUDGETING CONSIDERATIONS

WHP program developers should determine budgetary needs based on the types of resources required for a new or existing program. Table 3.2 presents a sample proportionate budget for an on-site fitness center. In setting a budget, program planners need to distinguish between *variable* (operating) expense

Table 3.1   Direct Cost Items and Projected Benefits of a Sample Pre-Work Back Stretch Program

Cost item	Daily	Week	Month	Year
Program leader				
Time required (hrs.)	.25	1.25	5	60
Hourly wage	× $15.00	× 15.00	× 15.00	× 15.00
Personnel cost	$3.75	18.75	75.00	900.00

Note: Time required reflects an average of 15 minutes per day for the program facilitator to prepare the worksite and perform the stretching and flexibility routine.

Productivity				
Company time used for program hours	.083	.415	1.66	19.92
Employees average wage (hr.)	$13.50	13.50	13.50	13.50
Number of employees	300	300	300	300
Productivity cost	$336.00	1,680.00	6,723.00	80, 676.00

Total personnel and productivity costs $81,576

After the combined personnel and productivity costs are calculated, the next step is to calculate projected savings from the program. For example:

Projected savings (1 year impact)

Health care costs	
Number of employees	300
Company's back injury rate last year (15%)	× .15
Number of employees reporting back injury	45
Average cost per back injury claim	× $1,525
Total low back injury claim costs	$68,625
Productivity loss	
Number of disability days per back injury	4.5
Number of back injuries	× 45
Number of back injury disability days	202.5
Average productivity loss cost per day[1]	× $138.24
Total productivity loss cost per year	$27,994
Total health care and productivity loss costs	$96,549
Estimated impact of program (90%)[2]	× .90
Estimated cost-avoidance (benefit)	$86,894

[1]Based on average hourly compensation (wage of $13.50 and company-paid benefits of $3.78) multiplied by 8 hours (average workday).

[2]Based on selected findings reported in the professional literature.

items such as personnel wages and utilities and *fixed* expenses such as property taxes and equipment depreciation. Since new programs require greater start-up expenses for personnel salaries, staff training, facilities, equipment, and materials, you can use an **expense management grid** to evaluate financing options (see p. 37). In developing a customized grid for a particular worksite, first list the major expense categories for a specific program or activity across the top of the grid. Second, list specific options on the left side of the grid. Third, review the available literature, conduct a survey of the local market, or talk with other worksite health professionals to assist you in identifying major issues. Finally, use all this information to identify possible relationships on the grid. For example, results from a market survey may indicate that it is more time- and cost-effective to hire a local physical therapist to conduct low back seminars at a worksite rather than training an employee to run the sessions.

Since the direct worth of expense items varies from site to site, program planners should consider various options to determine the most efficient way to use specific resources. Some typical questions during this phase include the following:

- Is it more economical for in-house personnel to operate on-site facilities and programs compared to an outside (contract) firm? What is the cost difference?

- Is new equipment needed or will used equipment do? If used or leased equipment is suitable, what type of warranty can be obtained? How often will the equipment need to be replaced?

Table 3.2 A Sample Proportionate Budget for an On-Site Fitness Center		
	Percent of total budget	
Cost category	**1st year**	**2nd year**
A. *Personnel*		
Salaries and benefits	35-40%	35-40%
Training	1-5	1-5
B. *Facilities*[1]	10	0
C. *Utilities*[1]	0	0
D. *Fitness equipment*[2]		
E. *Materials and supplies* (office, postage, phone, awards, surveys)[3]	5-10	5-10
F. *Advertising*	5-10	10-15
G. *Maintenance*	5-10	5-10
H. *Other* (unanticipated)	1-5	1-5

[1]Assuming minor renovation is necessary in the first year.

[2]A new 20′ × 24′ facility without equipment costs approximately $35,000 ($50 to $70 per square foot).

[3]Replacement costs are about one-third the initial purchasing cost.

EXPENSE MANAGEMENT GRID

List the major expense categories for a specific program or activity across the top of the grid. Then list specific options on the left side of the grid. Third, review the available literature, conduct a survey of the local market, or talk with other worksite health professionals to assist you in identifying major issues. Finally, use all this information to identify possible relationships on the grid.

Major expense categories:

- Staff   - Equipment   - Maintenance   - Facilities   - Materials   - Advertising

Onsite expenses _____

Offsite expenses _____

Purchase new _____

Purchase used _____

Equipment donated _____

Services contracted _____

Services negotiated _____

Possible bid? _____

Services donated _____

Other (list) _____

- Will in-house staff have the time and skills to analyze health claims data as quickly, cost-effectively, and objectively as an outside firm?

- Will an in-house EAP be as appealing to employees as an external EAP?

- What kind of resources may exist at the local university to assist with WHP efforts?

INTEGRATED HEALTH MANAGEMENT

Recent studies on the organizational frameworks and cost-control efforts of many U.S. companies have shown a direct relationship between **integrated health management** and cost control. As a group, companies operating an integrated approach showed average health care cost increases of only 2.5 percent per year, about a third less than the national average. This decisive cost-control advantage enables these companies to invest more money in research and development, employee training, and pay hikes. Even small and midsize organizations can benefit from an integrated health management framework (as we'll see in chapter 8).

The overall success of an integrated health management framework depends largely on an organization's ability to do the following:

- develop health management goals that are realistic,

- employ health management personnel with the skills to achieve each goal,

- delegate appropriate personnel to specific goals, and

- establish an operational framework to enhance interpersonal and interdepartmental communication and teamwork.

An integrated health management approach offers employers the greatest opportunity to achieve their goals. For example, many companies have integrated their health promotion activities within a highly visible division such as the human resources (see figure 3.1) or benefits department to enhance its visibility, credibility, and administrative support. Such integration provides daily opportunities for personnel to communicate and work across tradi-

tional departmental lines to achieve key health management goals. For instance, say an occupational health nurse does a basic health screening on a new employee and detects poor low back flexibility. Based on this information, the nurse may

- decide to meet with the personnel or human resources manager to discuss appropriate job opportunities within the employee's capabilities;

- refer the new employee to an exercise specialist to improve flexibility, and/or

- encourage the new employee to participate in the company's pre-work back stretch and strengthening program.

These interventions can improve both the employee's low back health and a company's ability to avoid preventable injuries and accidents at the worksite.

An integrated approach, though increasing in popularity nationwide, can have its disadvantages as well, the main one involving autonomy. By its nature an integrated approach depends on teamwork and decision by committee. This can work well, but the decision-making process might break down if department representatives push their own agendas. When this occurs, department leaders might become frustrated over the inability to arrive at decisions in a timely manner. Many health program planners get discouraged at how little clout they have in an integrated approach. Despite the possible downside, integrated health management has been a success overall.

Once program planners have made key decisions about goal setting, funding and budgeting, and how to manage WHP programs, they are ready to prepare a proposal for management. Presenting the program proposal is a crucial stage in the planning phase. Present the proposal poorly and the plug may be pulled on the program before it ever has a chance to prove its value.

PRESENTING YOUR PROPOSAL

A health promotion program proposal should address a company's specific health management needs. Although every proposal will be different,

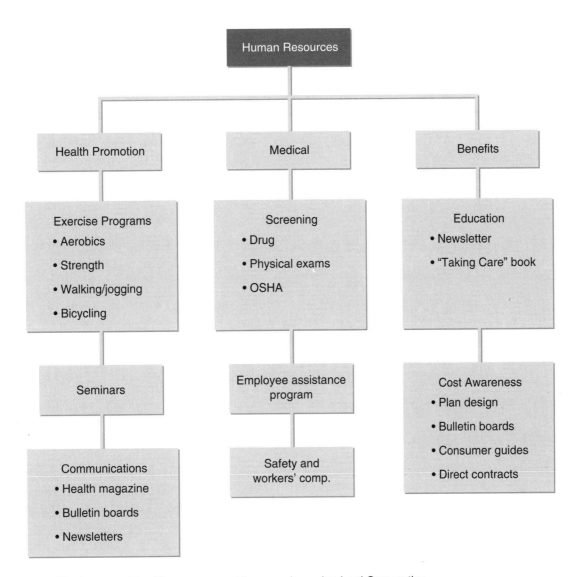

Figure 3.1 The integrated health management framework used at Lord Corporation.

each should contain most of the following sections:

- Problem identification
- Goal
- Environmental assessment
- Corporate strategies
- Resource assessment
- Proposed program
- Expected costs
- Expected benefits
- Overall benefit-cost projection

For example, assume that a company's health care costs are rising faster than anyone's projections and

that a health promotion program is being proposed. Upon reviewing the company's health care claims data, the task force discovers that (1) the most common type of health care claim filed by employees is *musculoskeletal* and (2) low back injuries are involved in most of these claims. Based on this information, the program planner prepares a proposal for a back injury prevention program (see pp. 40-42). Management will undoubtedly consider this proposal because it

1. clearly describes the identified problem,
2. suggests a particular program to address the problem, and
3. shows benefits will probably exceed programming costs.

PROGRAM PROPOSAL

A. Problem Identification

The task force reviewed the company's health care claims and cost data, which revealed the most common claims to be musculoskeletal:

Type	# of Claims	Total Cost	Average Cost/Claim
Back injuries	100	$65,000	$ 650
Knee injuries	33	9,174	278
Wrist injuries	14	1,400	100

B. Goal

To reduce the number and cost per claim of musculoskeletal injuries, especially low back injuries.

C. Environmental Assessment

Further analysis and worksite observations by on-site health personnel indicated the following:

• Employees most affected: 25- to 45-year-old men working in the shipping department.

• Most common time of occurrence: 75 percent of all low back injuries occurred in the first two hours of the work shift.

• Type of injury: 90 percent of all back injuries were classified as muscle strains in the low back.

• Activity at time of injury: 60 percent of all low back muscle strain injuries occurred while the victims were lifting.

D. Corporate Strategies

(What other organizations are doing to minimize back injuries) Task force members called local employers and reviewed several scientific journal articles on low back injury prevention programs. They found several companies with successful programs, such as the following:

Company	Program features	Impact
1. Biltrite Co. (Chelsea, MA)	Employee education Pre-work stretching	90% drop in workers' compensation
2. Capital Wire (Plano, TX)	Pre-work stretching Employee education	Fewer back injuries; $180,000 saved
3. Lockheed (Sunnyvale, CA)	Pre-work stretching Employee seminars	67.5% drop in total back injury costs

E. Resource Assessment

What types of on-site resources can be used to develop an effective low back injury prevention program? The task force coducted an on-site inventory that indicated:

• Available resources

  1. Facility: Large warehouse area

  2. Promotional materials: Employee newsletter

  3. Budget: $1,500 is available in the human resource department's discretionary fund

• Needed resources

  1. Equipment: Padded floor mats needed for back and abdominal floor exercises

  2. Incentives: A quarterly sweepstakes program with prizes!!!!!

(continued)

F. Proposed Program

Based on the health problem identified and resources available, the task force recommends the following program:

BACK BASICS

(A worksite back injury prevention program)

Target Area: Shipping department

Phase 1 (January): **Awareness and publicity.** The number of low back injuries reported at the worksite will appear in this month's issue of the employee newsletter and repeated on a quarterly basis. The issue will explain the primary reasons for the new program with specific responsibilities for shipping department supervisors, employees, and the occupational health nurse.

Phase 2 (February): **Training.** The occupational health nurse will conduct training sessions for all shipping supervisors and employees in predesignated team meetings. Topics will include back anatomy, ergonomic factors, and proper lifting and pulling/pushing techniques.

Phase 3 (March): **Incentives.** Worksite posters and newsletter articles will describe how to enter the Back Basics Sweepstakes program. All shipping department employees reporting no back injuries can compete for prizes at quarterly intervals (four times per year).

Phase 4 (March): **Implementation.** Shipping supervisors will lead their respective employee teams through a mandatory back stretch and strengthening routine during the first 5 minutes of their work shift; after the first week, employees will serve as team leaders on a rotating basis.

Phase 5 (July): **Monitoring and Evaluation.** The occupational health nurse will review back injury data every 6 months to determine the impact of the program. Results will be highlighted in the following newsletter.

G. Expected Costs

Based on the identification and needs assessment, the task force estimates that annual operating costs for the proposed program will be as follows:

1. Personnel: no additional cost
2. Facility: no additional costs (will use existing space)
3. Equipment: padded floor mats—$400
4. Promotions: sweepstakes prizes—$600

Total—$1,000

H. Expected Benefits

Based on a review of other worksite low back injury prevention programs, the following benefits are expected within 1 year of starting the program:

- Health care cost control
- Fewer job-related back injuries
- Fewer back injury claims
- Fewer back claims requiring compensation
- Reduced absenteeism

- Productivity enhancement
- Stronger stomach muscles
- Better back flexibility
- Better lifting capacity

(continued)

PROGRAM PROPOSAL *(CONTINUED)*

I. Overall Benefit-Cost Projection

The proposed program is modeled after successful worksite back injury prevention programs and expected to produce a minimum 10 percent impact. Thus the proposed program should reduce the number of expected low back injuries from 90 to 81. Since the average cost of one low back strain is about $1,000, a 10 percent impact would produce a cost savings of approximately $9,000. If two or more injuries are averted during the year, anticipated cost savings would exceed program costs, as shown in the table below:

Injuries avoided	Benefit	Program Cost	Benefit-Cost Ratio	Impact
9	$9,000	$1,000	9:1	Excellent
8	8,000	1,000	8:1	
7	7,000	1,000	7:1	Very good
6	6,000	1,000	6:1	
5	5,000	1,000	5:1	Good
4	4,000	1,000	4:1	
3	3,000	1,000	3:1	Fair
2	2,000	1,000	2:1	
1	1,000	1,000	1:1	Poor

Every proposal must meet these three criteria in order to be effective.

BREAK-EVEN ANALYSIS

While reviewing a proposal, management may want to know when a program or strategy will pay off or break even. For example, assume a company is planning to convert an old warehouse into a fitness center with a two-person staff consisting of a program director and a fitness specialist. By determining specific costs and usage patterns of the fitness center, program planners can develop a **break-even analysis.** A sample break-even analysis is shown on page 43.

In using any economic analysis technique, be aware that various factors can jeopardize expected outcomes. In our preceding example, the estimated timeframe of 4 years may be extended by unforeseen or uncontrollable events—if the participation level drops below the expected level; if participants miss an abnormal amount of work for reasons unrelated to exercise; or if employee wages and benefits or the company's cost to replace absent workers increase faster than absenteeism costs. On the other hand, if participation levels exceed the expected level, participant absenteeism drops, or wages and replacement costs increase more slowly than absenteeism costs, then the break-even point would occur earlier than 4 years.

Once the program has been proposed to and accepted by management, the program planner is nearly ready to implement the program. However, two more steps are necessary before the program can be safely launched: screening employees for health risks and giving the program a trial run.

EMPLOYEE HEALTH SCREENING

By providing WHP programs, an employer assumes a degree of risk. Legally, an employer may be held liable for an employee's injury if any of the following are true:

- An employee is injured while participating in a mandatory program or activity.

- The company benefits from the employee's attendance or participation in the program he or she is injured in.

- The employee is injured on the job.

Although WHP-related lawsuits are rare, worksites should take steps to minimize their liability risk. For example, many companies have positioned their programs so that workers' compensation insurance or private liability insurance will cover any program-related injuries.

BREAK-EVEN ANALYSIS FOR AN ON-SITE FITNESS CENTER FOR A MIDSIZE ORGANIZATION

Procedure

Determine fixed costs

a. Fitness center equipment: $20,060

b. Maintenance of equipment: $500

c. Depreciation of equipment: $500

Determine variable costs

a. Staffing (annual salaries)
   Program director: $30,000
   Fitness specialist: $25,000

b. Utilities, office materials, etc.: $4,000

c. Program advertising: $1,000

                    Total costs $81,060

Determine projected usage rate of fitness center

a. Size of workforce: 500 employees

b. Percentage of workforce × 15% (national
   expected to participate   avg.)

c. Usage rate: 75 employees

d. Number of weekly visits   × 2
   per participant

           Total weekly visits 150

Determine financial benefits from fitness center visits

The desired outcome will vary from program to program. The outcome used as the "benefit" in this example is *reduced absenteeism.*

a. Corporate benefit per participant: $2.76*

b. Number of total weekly participant   × 150
   visits

      Total corporate benefit per week $414
      (cost savings due to avoided absences)

*Based on research studies showing exercisers are absent at least 1.2 days less than non-exercisers; 1.2 days × $240" = $288 per absence; $288 ÷ 52 weeks = $5.53 ÷ 2 (weekly visits) = $2.76.

**Based on the U.S. worker's average wage and benefits of $15 per hour; 15 × 8 hours = $120; $120 paid each to the absent employee and a replacement = $240.

Determine break-even point by dividing total costs by financial benefit per week

a. Total costs (fixed and variable): $81,060

divided by

b. Corporate benefit per week $414

c. Time of participation needed   195.7 weeks
   to break even

Plot costs and benefits on a time frame (see figure 3.2)

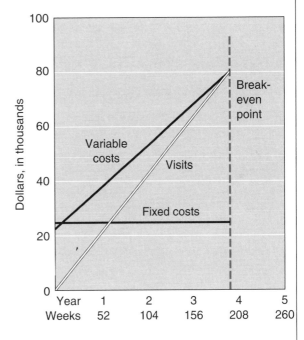

Figure 3.2   A sample break-even analysis.

Based on the preceding break-even analysis, the company's fitness center investment will pay for itself in 196 weeks (within 4 years).

A screening program that identifies high-risk employees for appropriate referral into specific programs can be an excellent strategy. However, organizations that have health and fitness or recreation facilities with admission or participation policies that would exclude or limit certain individuals from program activities should carefully review the requirements of the **Americans With Disabilities Act** (ADA). For example, using safety screening criteria is probably permissible under the Act, provided the criteria are based on actual risks, not stereotypical ones. The Americans With Disabilities Act (ADA) of 1990 stipulates that employers with 15 or more employees cannot discriminate on the basis of a person's disability. For printed information on the Act, contact the Publications Distribution Center at 1-800-669-3362. Worksites that use a screening system to admit or exclude individuals to exercise or recreation programs may have to modify their policies to accommodate the provisions of the law and should seek legal advice for guidance in reviewing current policies.

Also, health professionals responsible for developing and administering health screening protocols should comply with the following standards:

• Screening techniques should be medically warranted and conducted only by authorized, competent professionals.

• Before employees are screened, they should be informed of the purpose of the screening and any other pertinent information.

• Postscreening should be conducted in order for program personnel to interpret screening results to employees on an individualized basis.

• Screening should not rely solely on a physical exam to evaluate a person's total health status. A physical should identify organic signs and symptoms, such as high blood pressure or a heart murmur, but lifestyle habits and family history should also be reviewed during a health screen.

Virtually all employees have some level of measurable health risk. Several worksite studies indicate the following range:

Percentage of employees	Health risk level	Number of risk factors
5 to 20%	Low	0–1
30 to 60%	Moderate	2–3
5 to 20%	High	4–5
1 to 3%	Very high	6+

Because risk level varies so much, have screening procedures to detect risk factors in all employees who may participate in the WHP program. Any selected procedure should factor in age, gender, current health status, family history, activity level, health education interests, and occupation.

Traditional screening techniques may cost less than some contemporary methods, but the newer, more expensive techniques might be better at revealing problems. For example, when estimating heart disease risk, measuring the *ratio of total cholesterol-to-HDL cholesterol* level is more accurate, though slightly more expensive, than simply measuring total cholesterol. In most cases the extra cost of administering the more expensive screening technique is more than offset by the long-term savings of preventing an injury or a heart attack.

Since employee health risks vary across worksites, several different screening techniques should be considered. For example, one large-scale study conducted in a major medical center determined the cost-effectiveness of various screening techniques on a population demographically similar to that of America's workforce. One thousand adults were subjected to 10 different health-screening techniques to determine their validity and reliability. Listed from least expensive per problem detected to most expensive per problem detected, the five most cost-effective techniques were

1. health risk appraisal,

2. history and physical exam,

3. chem-12 (blood analysis),

4. urinalysis, and

5. CBC (complete blood count).

As cost-effective a screening tool as it is, **health risk appraisal** (HRA) cannot identify all health problems and should be used in conjunction with other screenings. For example, many worksites supplement a person's health/medical history with an HRA. In all situations, HRAs should be distributed and maintained only by authorized personnel. Otherwise, some employees may perceive that management could use certain types of information (alcohol intake, cigarette smoking, and current health problems, for example) as a basis for discrimination or dismissal.

In many worksites, in-house health management personnel conduct fitness screenings on employees. Unfortunately, some employees fail to show up for this important screening, which is often time consuming and labor intensive. One way to minimize "no-shows" is to first ask employees to complete the appropriate questionnaire, omitting the biomedical section. Screening personnel then review the questionnaires to identify employees who are not

"high risk" and permit them to enter the program. After participating in several sessions, employees are called in individually for biomedical measurements. Employees failing to attend the minimum number of sessions do not receive the biomedical screening until they do so.

PRE-EXERCISE SCREENING

Before employees enter an exercise, fitness, or recreation program, they should be thoroughly screened and cleared for participation. A **pre-exercise screening protocol** based on an employee's age and known risk factors is illustrated in figure 3.3.

Diagnostic laboratory testing is indicated if CHD risk factors include hyperlipidemia (high blood fats), hyperglycemia (high blood sugar), or hyperuricemia (blood in urine).

In developing a pre-exercise screening protocol, health professionals should remember that exercise

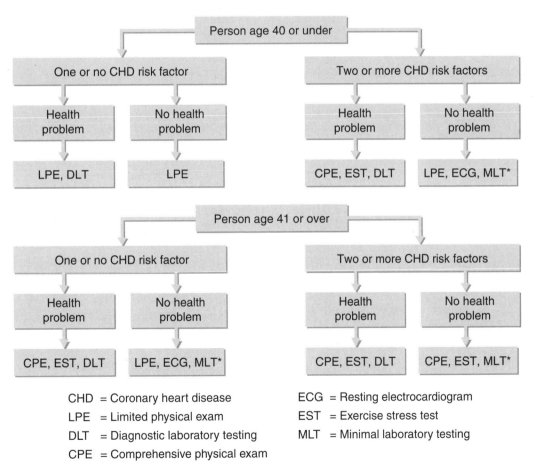

CHD = Coronary heart disease
LPE = Limited physical exam
DLT = Diagnostic laboratory testing
CPE = Comprehensive physical exam

ECG = Resting electrocardiogram
EST = Exercise stress test
MLT = Minimal laboratory testing

Figure 3.3 A sample pre-exercise screening protocol.

stress testing in a symptom-free population may detect more "false positives" than true positives. A **false positive** means that the test results indicate that something is wrong when in fact there is nothing wrong. Moreover, an exercise ECG has limited value in detecting or predicting coronary artery disease in asymptomatic persons with no known risk factors.

GXTs and Submaximal Tests

There are two types of pre-exercise tests: (1) symptom-limited, ECG-monitored, graded exercise tests (**GXTs**) and (2) **submaximal tests**.

GXTs should be conducted in a clinical setting by trained personnel under a physician's direct supervision. The GXT protocol, administered to the subject on a motorized treadmill, is specifically designed to detect coronary ischemia (a condition where the heart muscle receives insufficient oxygen due to diseased or blocked coronary arteries), and to determine functional capacity and safety of exercise for at-risk and symptomatic persons. Individuals at such risk and in need of the GXT protocol include persons who exhibit one or more of the following risk factors:

- Cigarette smoking
- Diabetes mellitus
- Family history of high blood cholesterol or heart disease
- Obesity
- High blood pressure (systolic over 160, diastolic over 90)
- Other high-risk condition as defined by a physician

Submaximal testing is used to determine an employee's fitness level and to assist in prescribing the right amount of exercise. A submaximal test can be administered with a bicycle ergometer, which is considerably less expensive than a motorized treadmill. To determine the appropriate testing protocol for each employee, check with a professional association such as the American College of Sports Medicine (ACSM) or the American Heart Association (AHA). In all cases, the selected protocol should be scientifically based and tailored to each individual's overall health status. For example, a common approach is to group employees into the following classes for pre-exercise screening purposes.

- Class I—Healthy, conditioned individuals of all ages
- Class II—Healthy, inactive individuals under age 35
- Class III—Healthy, inactive individuals over age 35
- Class IV—Conditioned individuals of all ages with major coronary risk factors, cardiovascular disease, or both
- Class V—Inactive individuals of all ages with major coronary risk
- Class VI—Inactive individuals of all ages with either acute or chronic cardiovascular disease
- Class VII—Individuals for whom exercise is contraindicated

Employees in classes I, II, or III should have the submaximal test. Those in all other classes should have the symptom-limited GXT. Employees in class VII may not be tested at all.

Other Risk and Liability Management Strategies

Employers are ultimately responsible for the safety of their WHP programs and must minimize the prospect of participants' injuries. Before they enter any type of company-sponsored exercise program, employees should be informed in writing of their personal responsibility in meeting all pre-exercise clearance requirements. Most companies require employees to complete an Informed Consent Form before participating. However, for maximum protection, employers should develop clear and concise policies requiring each participant to read such releases in the presence of a staff member and to acknowledge his or her understanding in writing. Without such documentation, an employee may claim that he or she signed the release unwittingly. Legal counsel should be consulted in developing and reviewing all informed consent and liability release forms.

See figure 3.4 for a sample Informed Consent Form that you can modify for your needs. Additional risk management guidelines include:

- Making sure all exercise instructors, supervisors, and program directors are properly certified by a reputable organization

---

Informed Consent Form

In consideration of my voluntary participation in [organization's name] health promotion program or any other activities sponsored by [organization] conducted on or off [organization's] property, I hereby release and discharge [organization] from any and all claims for damages suffered by me as a result of my participation in these activities. I specifically release and discharge [organization] and its health promotion staff from all injuries or damages arising from or contributing to any physical impairment or defect I may have, whether latent or patent, and agree that [organization] is under no obligation to provide physical examination or other evidence of my fitness to participate in such activities, these being my sole responsibility. Further, I understand that participation is not a condition of employment at [organization].

Date _____ Signature _____

(For Office Use Only)

Employee health status

____ Excellent

____ Good

____ Fair

____ Poor

____ Very poor

Pre-activity screenings

Type	Date	Staff	Results
____	____	____	____
____	____	____	____
____	____	____	____

Activity recommendation

____ Approved for participation

____ Approved, conditional

____ Rejected, further screening necessary

Program Director _____ Date _____

Figure 3.4 A sample informed consent form.

- Requiring all participants in high-risk activities to wear appropriate clothing and use appropriate equipment

- Making sure all equipment and facilities such as spas, whirlpools, steam rooms, and tanning salons feature clear, easy-to-see instructions with precautionary warnings

- Explaining the possibility of injuries associated with aerobics, racquetball, weight lifting, and other activities to all employees before they participate

- Requiring participants to sign an Informed Consent Form prior to participating

- Using only nationally recognized screening tests and procedures

- Developing and following a reliable accident reporting system

- Developing a hierarchy of supervision to ensure accountability for all phases of the program

- Designating who is responsible to whom and for what specific duties

For additional information on liability issues related to health screening, consult *Exercise Standards and Malpractice Reporter* and *The Sports, Parks, and Recreation Law Reporter*. For more information, write the Professional Reports Corporation, 4571 Stephen Circle, N.W., Canton, Ohio, 44718 or call 216-499-0200.

Many smaller worksites do not have adequate personnel, facilities, and equipment to conduct appropriate pre-exercise testing. In such settings, a questionnaire can be used to assess a person's cardiovascular health. Employees with *any* positive

CARDIOVASCULAR SCREENING QUESTIONNAIRE		
Condition	Yes	No
1. Have you ever had a heart attack?	___	___
2. Have you ever had a heart problems?	___	___
3. Have you ever had "angina" (chest pain)?	___	___
4. Were you born with a heart condition?	___	___
5. Have you ever had high blood pressure?	___	___
6. Have you ever had diabetes?	___	___
7. Do you smoke?	___	___
8. Have you ever had a thyroid condition?	___	___
9. Have you ever had surgery in the past?	___	___
10. Are you currently taking any medication?	___	___
11. If you're female, are you pregnant?	___	___

Figure 3.5 A sample cardiovascular screening questionnaire.

responses on the questionnaire should meet with their personal physicians for further consultation and permission to exercise. You may use the questionnaire shown in figure 3.5 or modify it as necessary.

Because health screening is both labor- and time-intensive, efficiency is particularly important for small businesses. Although most small businesses do not have in-house screening personnel, they can consider networking with local agencies by

• negotiating with the local health department to conduct a basic health screening for employees at little or no cost;

• inviting representatives from local health clubs to conduct complimentary employee health screenings in exchange for an opportunity to advertise their services at the worksite;

• joining other small businesses in sponsoring a health fair for employees and their families;

• inviting local health associations and health care providers to provide health screenings; or

• asking trained faculty members (exercise physiologists, physical educators, nurses, physical therapists, and health educators) at a local university to conduct employee health screenings in exchange for using their worksite as a possible research site.

BUILDING EVALUATION INTO YOUR PROGRAM

Some WHP program planners make the mistake of designing an evaluation *after* the health promotion program is underway rather than during the planning phase. This often leads to rushed evaluation procedures that yield unreliable results. Because crafting the evaluation is so important, chapter 5 is devoted to that subject. Study the information you find there carefully, as proper evaluation planning at this stage is essential for the program to fulfill its potential.

MATCHING GOALS AND PROGRAMS

Assuming appropriate goals have been set in the first place (see p. 34 for discussion of goal setting), the best way to evaluate a program's success is to compare the program's results to the program's goals. Unfortunately, results cannot be judged until after the program has been completed. Since evaluation procedures need to be set up early, we need ways to anticipate realistic results of a program. Two good ways to predict the impact of health promotion programs are to (1) talk to other WHP professionals who have implemented similar programs and (2) review the literature to see what types of programs have had a positive influence. For instance, reviewing the tabular data below from published studies on WHP should help you know what to expect from a given program and thereby help you set standards to evaluate your own program.

Program	Short-term variables (less than 2 years)	Long-term variables (2 years or more)
Consumer education	Self-care practices	Health care usage/costs
	Cost-awareness	
Exercise	Health-related absenteeism	Health care and usage/costs
	Accidents	Turnover
	Attitude toward self, employer, and work	
	Physical and mental	
	Health/performance	
	Productivity	
Employee assistance program (EAP)	Absenteeism	Health care usage
	Accidents	Turnover
	Productivity	
	Attitude toward self, employer, and work	
	Physical and mental health	
	Return to work	
High blood pressure control	Blood pressure	Health care usage
	Physical health	
Back	Low back injuries	Disability and workers' compensation claims
	Productivity	
	Severity of injury and costs	
	Recovery and return to work	
Medical self-care	Health care usage	
	Health care costs	
Nutrition and weight control	Physical and mental health	Health care usage
Smoking cessation	Physical health	Absenteeism
	Property insurance	Health insurance
	Product	Life insurance
	Property damage and depreciation	Premature death
Stress management	Coping skills	Health care usage
	Physical health	Health care costs
Worklife	Attitude toward employer	
	Quality of work performed	
	Productivity	

Variables that relate directly to employee health are called **employee health indicators.** Variables closely related to an organization's health and performance are called **organizational health indicators.** Here is a sampling of each category:

Employee health indicators	Organizational health indicators
Blood pressure	Absenteeism
Body fat percentage	Accidents and injuries
Body weight	Health care utilization (claims)
Cholesterol level	Health care costs
Flexibility	Productivity
Heart rate	Turnover
Coping skills (stress)	Workers' compensation costs
Eating habits	
Safety belt usage	
Substance use	
Tobacco use	

Some indicators are influenced by a company's operations and record-keeping practices. Take absenteeism, for example. Many companies classify absences as either controllable or uncontrollable. Some typical examples of both classifications:

Controllable/ unscheduled	Uncontrollable/ scheduled
Due to poor health/illness	Jury duty
Falsely calling in "sick"	Maternity/paternity leave
Faking an injury	Attending a funeral
Work-related disability	Inclement weather

Since WHP programs have no impact on uncontrollable factors, program goals and evaluation procedures will focus on controllable variables. See chapter 5 for a complete discussion of evaluation procedures.

GIVING THE PROGRAM A TRIAL RUN

As the planning process winds down and the program nears implementation, it's a good idea to conduct a trial run to identify potential problems and make necessary adjustments. This is especially good when planning a new exercise program or facility in order to assess traffic flow, space, equipment, facilities, and employee interest. A trial run can be conducted in four steps:

1. Recruit the number of employees you expect to participate at one time.
2. Explain the structure and purpose of the exercise facility and equipment and how to use the apparatus
3. Have each person occupy a specific piece of equipment so that the entire facility is occupied.
4. Instruct all participants to exercise at their stations for a set time before proceeding to the next station.

As these steps are undertaken, check to see if the time allotted is enough for employees to complete each routine at each station. Is the transition smooth or choppy? If there is a delay, identify possible reasons and consider revising the facility layout or instructions for better efficiency.

This stage is a good time for program planners to confirm program goals, procedures, personnel responsibilities, resource requirements, and suggested implementation and completion dates for the program. A sample framework is illustrated in figure 3.6.

Planning and Implementation Format

Major Goals:

1. Reduce the number of low back injuries to warehouse workers.

2. Reduce the cost per low back injury.

3. Encourage employees to practice prework low back stretching and strengthening routines on a daily basis.

Procedure: Design and implement on-site strategies to promote new low back program: (a) meet with corporate communication department to discuss promotional options; design program logo and script; (b) inform supervisors of new program and how they can promote it; (c) distribute brochures to supervisors; place posters at key sites; (d) distribute program announcements in paycheck stuffers.

Resources	Facilities	Personnel assigned	Timeline	Outcome measure
Brochure	At work stations	Health promotion specialist (a, b, c)	Design by Jan. 15	Number of injuries; cost per injury; number of participants
Posters	In warehouse		Under way by Feb. 15	
Paycheck stuffers		Program assistant (c)		
		Personnel department (d)		

Figure 3.6   A Sample Planning and Implementation Format.

What Would You Do?

Suppose you work for a company that has never had WHP. Management has asked you to design and implement a new medical self-care program for employees. Your research efforts show that the most effective intervention is voluntary and consists of on-site seminars, self-care books, and financial incentives. You learn that this program can yield as much as a $4 benefit for every $1 spent. However, it appears at least 50 percent of employees must participate in the program for at least a year for this positive benefit-cost ratio to be achieved. Your worksite is currently downsizing, and management expects you to show the $4-to-$1 return rate within 6 months. In preparing your proposal for the new program, what should you do to achieve management's goal within the shorter timeframe? Should you propose a mandatory program to ensure 100 percent participation? If not, should you recommend higher financial incentives? Should you offer a higher number of on-site seminars? What would you do? Describe and justify your strategy.

IMPLEMENTING WORKSITE HEALTH PROGRAMS

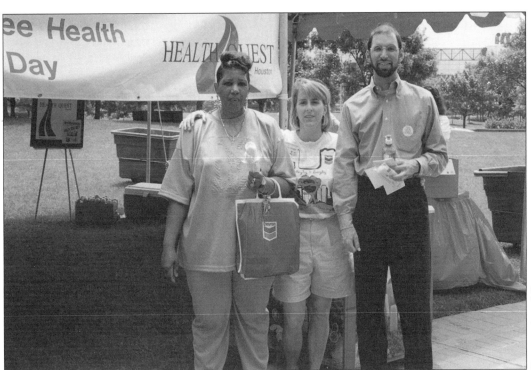

Photo courtesy of Chevron

Some of America's most successful WHP programs do not have expensive facilities, a large staff, or a hefty budget. However, an ingredient that most of these programs do share is a program director who is committed to identifying needs, coordinating responsibilities, and applying resources toward achieving reasonable, well-defined goals. Below is a checklist that includes a dozen features you'll typi-cally find in WHP programs developed and run by such directors. Program planners may copy and use the checklist to see how well their programs meet the criteria.

Of course, developing a program that includes all 12 of these features requires careful planning prior to the program's implementation along with regular maintenance once the program is underway.

CHECKLIST FOR A SUCCESSFUL PROGRAM

Choose those items that are true for your program. If you check fewer than 10, you may have more work to do.

_____ 1. Top management supports the program.

_____ 2. The company has a designated budget for health promotion.

_____ 3. The program is free or inexpensive.

_____ 4. Qualified personnel operate the program.

_____ 5. The program staff seeks regular input from both management and employees.

_____ 6. Opportunities to participate in the program are convenient for all employees.

_____ 7. The program director conducts health screenings and staff surveys to monitor interest in the program and follows up accordingly.

_____ 8. Attractive and informative program materials are available for employees to take home.

_____ 9. When possible, health promotion activities are open to dependents and retirees.

_____ 10. The company's mission statement cites a healthy workforce among its top priorities.

_____ 11. The program provides both general and customized health promotion activities for employees at all work locations.

_____ 12. The company gets involved in local health promotion programs to show its commitment to improving the community's health status.

Plans for launching the program include (1) developing a strategy to make the program enticing to employees—that is, a **marketing strategy**—and (2) coming up with ideas for maintaining participation in the program once it's up and running.

DEVELOPING A MARKETING STRATEGY

Marketing is defined in *Webster's* as "an aggregate of functions involved in moving goods from producer to consumer." Depending on the goods involved, these functions might include describing the product to those who have never heard of it; explaining what the product is and how to use it; advertising the product so that consumers know it exists; monitoring the product at the manufacturing site to check for consistent quality; distributing the product in various quantities to match the needs of different consumer segments; transporting the product to places where the consumer can easily get to it; again monitoring the product at the distributor, wholesaler, or retailer to ensure consistent quality; and seeking feedback about the product from the

consumer to learn ways to improve the product's future marketability. When people talk about "goods," we tend to think of tangible items, but the marketing principles that apply to tangibles also apply to intangibles such as WHP. As the product's "producer," the program director's job is to make the product available and appealing to the "consumer"—in this case company employees.

Organizations such as Johnson & Johnson, PepsiCo, Coors, and Union Pacific Railroad manage WHP in the same way they approach marketing their primary products and services: by focusing on the four Ps—Product, Price, Placement, and Promotion, also called the "marketing mix."

PRODUCT

When your product is health promotion—helping people to feel better and live longer—you might think the product would sell itself, but unfortunately this is not the case. As with all other products or services, a health promotion program must be marketed in such a way that consumers find it attractive and worth experiencing. As summarized in "The four Ps of Marketing" on page 55, important questions to ask about the program include, What is our service? Is it tangible, visible, or measurable? What is

THE FOUR PS OF MARKETING

Questions to Address	Considerations

Product
1. What is our product or service?
2. Is it tangible, visible, and measurable?
3. What is the employee (or client) need for the product or service:
  • To look better?
  • To feel better?
  • To be more productive?
  • To reduce health risks?
  • To socialize with others?
	Define the product or service in precise terms.

Price 1. Should we charge participants? 2. Can the employee/company reasonably afford the product? 3. Does the product or service produce a greater benefit than cost? See page 72 in chapter 5 for an overview of benefit-cost analysis.	Cost may be an extremely important factor in small businesses and other organizations with tight budgets. Thus, variously priced options of the product or service may be necessary. Determine the probable cost savings of the product or service.

Placement
1. Who will receive the product or service?
  • All employees?
  • High-risk employees?
  • Only men or only women?
2. What employees could benefit from the product or service?
	Consider breaking the workforce into segments based on specific attributes:
	  • Age • Division or department
	  • Gender • Past participation status
	  • Family size • Work shift
	  • Type of work • HRA respondents
	  • Educational level • Commuting time to/from work

Promotion
1. What types of incentives can be used to make the product or service?
	A demonstrated benefit must be shown for consumers to use the product or service. Use tangible incentives to create a unique selling point. Some examples include:
	  • Freebies (T-shirts, child care, health screenings) • Discounts or rebates (health insurance, memberships, etc.)
	  • Personalized training or counseling

2. What is the best time to promote the product or service?	Periods of high unemployment, sluggish business, or merger talks may preoccupy or obligate some employees to work overtime and thus not respond to the product or service.
3. Where should promotional efforts be implemented?	Consider on-site and off-site options (direct mailings to employees' homes, company newsletter, bulletin boards, e-mail, benefits updates, paycheck stuffers, voice mail).
4. What promotional techniques are most effective?	

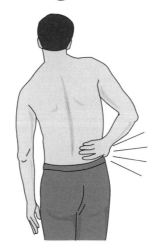

Health Committee Members: — Promotion
Please Post on all Bulletin Boards

— Product

GET BACK TO HEALTH

Are you tired of sore back muscles and back aches?
Want more energy for life?
Then, it's time to get back to health!

Placement —

For anyone concerned about their back

Price — **Free!** — Unique selling point

All participants receive a free back screening

Monday, November 25th
Conference Room #14
4:30–5:30 PM

- -

Sign-Up Form

Name ——————————— Dept.———————

Reason for attending program

———————————————————————

Please return form to Health & Safety Office
by November 1st. *Thank you!*

Figure 4.1   A sample low back program promotion poster highlighting the four Ps of the marketing mix.

the need for this service? Employees need to know precisely what they are being offered. Does the WHP program require an hour-a-day commitment or only an hour a week? Does the program take a hands-on or a hands-off approach? How much flexibility is there for employees with busy schedules outside of work? Can they participate in the program during work hours? What exactly can they gain by participating in a program that promotes health? Will gains be financial, tangible, practical, or otherwise directly applicable to their current situation, or will they be more abstract and hard to measure? These questions and many more must be answered to employees' satisfaction if they are going to be enticed to try the program.

PRICE

No matter how the program's expenses are covered—100 percent by the employer, 100 percent by the employee, or somewhere in between—employees must understand that the benefits of the program outweigh their own personal costs or they will not participate. Even if a program is free of charge in terms of money, some employees may find it too expensive in terms of time. Whether the costs are in dollars, hours, or ounces of sweat, the employees' perception must be that they have more to gain than they have to lose.

Of course there are price considerations from the company's perspective as well. Many companies will find that a program is not financially feasible unless it is funded in part by participants. Will this mean employees will avoid the program? Will they resent paying even a small percentage and consequently choose not to participate? Such questions need answers before the program is launched.

PLACEMENT

Another consideration for WHP program directors and their companies is which employees to focus on when starting the program. Should the program target all employees equally, or should only particular groups be targeted? Keep in mind that success or failure is often determined in the early stages of any endeavor. If the program is to receive a trial run, it might be best to include only some employees rather than all, as this way if the trial fails the program can be adjusted and restarted without losing credibility with all employees. If all employees are targeted and the first run of the program fails, it will be more difficult to create enthusiasm again.

Some WHP programs aim at only high-risk employees, as these often are the ones who can benefit most. However, it's also true that some high-risk employees are less likely to participate in a WHP program than regular-risk or low-risk employees are. Why is this? Part of the reason is explained under the Price section above: some workers simply feel that their cost in time or exertion is not worth the benefits they will receive from the program. The same factors that have led to their being high risk make them less likely to sacrifice time and effort for health improvements. On the other hand, the employees who are at relative low risk because they value fitness will be more likely to participate in a WHP program, as the program is aligned with their current values. Such considerations, though potentially disheartening for program directors, need to be acknowledged and dealt with if the program is to have realistic goals and successful methods of countering potential pitfalls.

It can be worthwhile to vary aspects of a WHP program for different groups of employees. If possible, a company might consider offering a *cafeteria* program in which employees pick the parts of the program that they perceive best suits them. For instance, instead of focusing on nutrition or stress management for all employees for a given week, a program might give employees the option to forego that week's emphasis and spend an additional week on quitting smoking instead.

Sometimes it can be advantageous to place employees into groups based on age, gender, type of work, or other factors. This allows individuals to focus on the areas they are most concerned about. For example, a group of 20- to 25-year-olds might require less aerobic training than a group of 35- to 45-year-olds, whereas the latter group might need less instruction regarding nutrition than the former group would need.

PROMOTION

Though health promotion has its own rewards, sometimes these rewards take too long for the impatient beginner. Many newcomers to a health or fitness program quit before they have gained any of the benefits they would have received if they had just stuck with the program 1 more month. Understanding this, WHP program directors usually offer external, tangible rewards for consistent participation in the first few weeks or months of the program. After that, external rewards are less necessary as participants begin to enjoy the more satisfying internal rewards of feeling better, increased self-esteem, reduced stress, and so on.

Early in the program the WHP director needs to decide what kind of external rewards work best. Are employees more likely to show up for a free Frisbee or T-shirt, or would they prefer passes to a health club or local theaters? This information can be learned from trial and error, of course, but a simpler way to identify popular incentives is to ask employees what types they prefer via an Incentive Survey (see chapter 2).

Again, nothing promotes a program better than demonstrated benefits in areas that employees care about. If a nutrition program helps workers lose weight and improve self-esteem, chances are good they will return for as long as the program provides these benefits. On the other hand, if employees do not see the benefits they are gaining in the program, they will need external incentives for adherence until the more important internal benefits are more clearly seen and felt.

SPECIFIC IDEAS FOR PROMOTING THE NEW PROGRAM

At the beginning of the chapter we presented a checklist with a dozen features common to successful WHP programs. Worksites vary tremendously, so there are no guarantees, but if a WHP program director can check at least 10 of the 12 items on the checklist, he or she can rest assured that it is a quality program that should win popularity among participants. If the director checks fewer than 10 of the items, the program may need to be modified in ways that help the program better resemble those programs that have proven themselves successful.

If a program contains 10 or more of the dozen features, it is probably ready to be implemented at the worksite. Here are important tips for program directors to keep in mind as they promote their new program:

• When possible, programs should be offered on or near normal working hours and on the days and times preferred by employees.

• Program facilities should be available to workers on all shifts.

• When advertising the program, it is best to use a positive and catchy title for the program rather than a negative title. For instance, instead of referring to a nutrition program as "Weight Loss Program" use "Eating for the Good Life." Other examples: "Taking Charge!" (exercise program), "Take Over Time" (stress-management program), "Kicking Butts" (smoking cessation program).

• Personal testimonies presented by previous program participants highlight the benefits of participating in the program. To be the most inspirational, these testimonies should be short and to the point.

• New participants can be charged a small fee ($5) that is pooled for reimbursing employees who reach their personal goals.

• One way of winning over stubborn holdouts is to offer a sweepstakes or lottery to all program newcomers.

• Employees should have at least one hour of paid release time each week to participate in on-site health programs.

• One-on-one or small group (interdepartmental) competitions provide motivation and fun for participants.

• Offering 50 percent of the company's healthcare cost savings to program participants is a good way to show sincere interest in the needs of employees.

PROGRAM ADHERENCE

Once a program has been successfully promoted and is underway, program planners need strategies for motivating employees to stick with the program. Many employees are gung-ho at the beginning but lose interest if they don't see immediate results for their efforts. Since perceptible changes in health and fitness are often slow in coming, it can help to offer other, external, rewards until the internal reward of feeling better becomes a major factor in program adherence. Below are some other recommendations for helping employees stay with a program. (Note that extrinsic rewards may be more effective if they are offered only after the initial momentum has slowed.)

• Help employees set realistic goals. Break a long-term goal into short-term goals (e.g., split a proposed 40-pound weight loss into four monthly goals of losing 10 pounds per month).

• Stress the need to start out slowly, especially in exercise and weight loss.

• Give regular verbal support and written feedback to all participants while assessing progress.

• Establish a point system and offer "wellness bucks" to redeem for mugs, T-shirts, self-care books, and other prizes.

• Use a map to signify the distance covered by participants in a coast-to-coast "cross-country challenge"—give awards at certain landmarks or cities.

• Feature a "participant of the month" for outstanding attendance or performance.

• Sponsor a fun run/walk with participants predicting their finishing time; reward those with the closest actual times.

• Use an honor system to reward employees who promote their health at home and on the road.

For example, create personal health promotion checksheets for specific topics (exercise, nutrition, weight loss, smoking cessation). Have employees check off their weekly accomplishments and submit them at regular intervals for prizes (see figure 4.2).

END-OF-PROGRAM REWARDS

As a program nears completion, WHP planners should be thinking ahead to the next program. Part of this involves motivating employees who have finished one program to continue with others that will be of benefit to them. Here are some suggested rewards to give those employees who complete a program:

• Enter the employee in a sweepstakes or lottery. Draw one or more winners.

Table 4.1   Sample Personal Health Promotion Checksheet

Instructions: Calculate points earned for each week and the entire month. Turn the checksheet in to your supervisor by the first day of each month. Point credits are as follows:

15 minutes of nonstop activity = 2 points
20 minutes of nonstop activity = 3 points
25 minutes of nonstop activity = 4 points
30 minutes of nonstop activity = 5 points
35+ minutes of nonstop activity = 6 points

	Type of exercise completed					
Week number	Walking	Biking	Swimming	Jog-running	Other (list)	Total points
1	2	3				
	2	3				
	2	3				15
2		3				
			3			
	2					
	2					10
3	3					
	3	2				
		4				12
4	4					
		4				
	2					10
					Monthly total: 47	

- Print the employee's photo in the company's newsletter.

- Designate a "wall of fame" to highlight employees who finished a program.

- Offer the employee with the greatest improvement the "most valuable participant" parking space.

- Give away program-specific T-shirts after the final session (e.g., "I Kicked Butts" at the end of the smoking-cessation program).

- Ask management to send a congratulatory letter to employees who complete a program.

ATTRACTING NONPARTICIPANTS AND HIGH-RISK EMPLOYEES

While incentives and rewards work well at some worksites, all companies have their share of nonparticipants. Such "no-shows" are costly, as they often have greater health risks than participants do and thus incur more health care services in the long run. At least three large-scale studies conducted on employees at Ceridian Corporation, Steelcase Corporation, and Chrysler Corporation show that workers with potentially modifiable risk factors (e.g., smoking, obesity, and inactivity) are absent more and incur greater health care expenses than lower risk employees. Presumably, these individuals could benefit from WHP activities—yet fewer than 5 percent of all high-risk employees participate in WHP programs.

As more companies become aware of the correlation between health status and health care expense, they are appealing to the hard-to-reach sector by offering customized incentives and rewards. However, to be successful, program planners first need to identify various segments of a workforce to determine their particular interests and dispositions.

A typical work force may consist of four (or more) segments. The first group is often called the "diehards" because of their strong interest and regular participation in worksite and community-based health programs. These employees are the easiest to recruit and will often assist in various capacities (e.g., serve as a fitness leader).

The second segment of the work force are those employees who express "an interest" in their health but often need tangible incentives and regular encouragement from family members, co-workers, and

staff members to begin and adhere to a health program.

A third segment, perhaps best called the "conditionals," *might* participate if the conditions are personally appealing, such as a free program on company time. They also prefer to participate with a buddy or in a group with their immediate co-workers.

A fourth segment, the "resisters," is the toughest group to motivate for worksite participation. These employees have little interest in their personal health and often delay lifestyle changes until a major crisis such as a heart attack has occurred. Unfortunately, many resisters have never had a healthy lifestyle and thus cannot appreciate the many benefits of good health.

There's no secret recipe for motivating the resisters—which doesn't mean that program planners should not continue to try to get these employees involved. However, the good news is that a WHP program *can* be successful without signing up every employee. In most cases the success or failure of a program will depend on customized promotional campaigns and programs that center on employees' likes, dislikes, and capabilities. Using interest surveys and other assessment tools (see chapter 2) can help staff members plan appealing programs. Of course, carefully targeted incentives and rewards that fit individual and group preferences offer the greatest potential. However, promotional strategies that include awareness and hands-on activities should not be discounted.

DEVELOPING A HEALTH FAIR

One of the best ways to generate employee awareness and participation is a worksite health fair that includes colorful exhibits, audiovisual displays, educational materials, and various health screenings.

RECRUITING PARTICIPANTS

Program planners should ask selected employees to assist in setting up exhibits or distributing handouts for the fair. Finding volunteers may be easier if management allows employees to help on company time; however, many employees (the die-hards) will be willing to volunteer under any circumstances. Interest in participating in a health fair is usually high among community groups in which good health is valued. The following organizations or individuals should be invited to participate.

- County health department
- Fire, rescue, and police departments
- Local hospitals
- Medical, dental, and nursing auxiliaries
- Private optometrists and chiropractors
- Representatives from the American Heart Association, American Lung Association, American Cancer Society, and other reputable organizations
- College or university faculty and students in health-related disciplines

After receiving a verbal agreement from an organization or individual, it's important to seal the commitment by following up in writing. This letter will also serve as a notice to all who participate that the health fair is nonprofit and that the company holding the fair will not accept responsibility for losses or damages incurred during the fair. To avoid any possible legal problems, the company's WHP director will need to receive a signed copy of the letter from all participants. A sample letter, shown on page 62, can be modified to suit the circumstances of the company holding the health fair.

A HEALTH FAIR PLANNING FRAMEWORK

When planning the worksite health fair, program planners need to consider their compiled data on employee needs and interests (collected through various techniques discussed in chapter 2). This information is helpful in progressing through the three phases of building a health fair: preliminary planning, development, and implementation.

PHASE I—PRELIMINARY PLANNING

1. Determine primary health fair goals.
2. Review and rank health needs using company health records (accident data, medical claims data, workers' compensation data).

3. Identify and assess on-site and community health resources.
4. Develop and distribute a survey to local health promotion and health care providers to determine their interest in participating in a health fair.
5. Compile survey information into a database showing providers' names, services, or products with cost figures, and each contact person's name, address, and phone number.

PHASE II—HEALTH FAIR DEVELOPMENT

1. Choose an on-site health fair coordinator.
2. Develop a theme and logo.
3. Set locations, dates, and times for the event.
4. Prepare a working budget.
5. Confirm participation with community providers.
6. Meet with all participants and exhibitors to discuss the health fair layout and individual requirements for setting up.
7. Design and prepare publicity materials (e.g., newsletter articles, flyers, and posters).
8. Ask management to write an endorsement letter to encourage employee participation.

PHASE III—PROGRAM IMPLEMENTATION

1. Contact all community providers and on-site personnel participants about final arrangements including setup and dismantling times and procedures.
2. Conduct a mock walk-through to check traffic flow, spacing, and supervision needs.
3. Open the fair!

PROMOTING THE FAIR

Posters, bulletin boards, newsletters, electronic mail, and other internal resources can be used to advertise the health fair and subsequent programs to employees. For greatest exposure, promotional materials should be displayed at key locations at least 2 weeks before the fair.

Timing is important. Many worksites launch health fairs in January to be in sync with employees' New Year's resolutions. Or planners might consider holding the fair in mid-May during the week

SAMPLE LETTER TO HEALTH FAIR PARTICIPANTS

Dear _____ :

(Health Promotion Exhibitor/Provider)

Thank you for expressing interest in our health fair, to be held on October 4–6. Participation by _____
_____ such as _____ will help make our event a huge success!

(individuals/organizations) (you/yours)

This letter confirms our arrangement for your participation in our _____.

(event name)

All of your activities at the fair [describe service: give a presentation, present an exhibit, provide a service], and the activities of your representative will be as an independent contractor of and not as an agent for or an employee of (client company).

[If contractor will be doing an invasive, diagnostic, or potentially risky procedure, include the next paragraph.]

_____ shall indemnify and hold _____,

(Contractor name) (client company)

and their respective agents and employees harmless from any and all manner of loss, whatsoever (including reasonable costs of litigation and attorneys' fees) which _____

(client company)

may hereafter incur, become responsible for, or pay out as a result of death or bodily injury to any person or destruction or damage to any property arising out of _____

(client company's)

negligence (or that of their respective agents and employees), or in connection with the services provided by Contractor, except to the proportionate extent that such loss, liability, damage or claim was due to the willful misconduct of _____, its respective agents and employees.

(client company)

[If the contractor will be doing an invasive, diagnostic, or potentially risky procedure or will be providing a piece of equipment on which trial uses will be offered, include the next paragraph.]

As an independent contractor, you are responsible for having current general and professional [include also "product" liability if the contractor is an equipment seller who is bringing in equipment which individuals will use] liability insurance coverage (minimum of $1,000,000). Please return with this lettter copies of the appropriate certificates of insurance.

[If the contractor is a sole proprietor or not affiliated with a large reputable organization, such as a local hospital, and if the service is an invasive, diagnostic, or potentially risky procedure, include the following paragraph.]

Please prepare an Informed Consent and Release of Liability form for individuals to sign before taking part in your service. _____ should be released from all liabilities associated

(Client company)

with your service. Enclose a copy of the form with your confirmation.

Your services will be provided at no charge to _____. [If individuals desiring

(client company)

service will pay, note fee schedule.] We are looking forward to the upcoming _____.

(event name)

We appreciate your role in making it a success. If you understand and agree to the above arrangements and requirements, sign in the space provided below. To participate in the health fair, the exhibitor must sign and return the original copy of this letter, along with any required documents named above by _____. If you have any questions about the above requests, please do not

(date)

hesitate to call me at _____.

(phone number)

Sincerely,

Acknowledged and agreed to by _____

Name (please print) _____ Date _____

Themes and Occasions for Promoting Health Fairs	
Theme	**Month**
Eye care	January
Dental health	February
Heart	
Wise health consumer	
Drug awareness week	Late February or early March
Nutrition	March
Cancer awareness	April
Alcohol awareness	
Child abuse prevention	
STD awareness	
Physical fitness and sports	May
National Health and Fitness Day	Mid-May
Arthritis	
Asthma and allergy awareness	
Improved hearing and speech	
High blood pressure awareness	
Mental health	
Dairy	June
Safety	
National nondependence day	July 4
Cholesterol awareness	August
Baby safety	
Cholesterol education	
Sickle-cell anemia	September
Breast awareness	
AIDS awareness	
Alcohol awareness week	
Crime prevention awareness	
Domestic violence awareness	
Communicating with your children	
Family health month	
Talk about prescriptions	
Mental illness awareness	November
Great American Smokeout	Mid-November
Domestic violence awareness	
Child safety and protection	
Diabetes awareness	
Home health care	
Drunk driving prevention	December

of National Employee Health and Fitness Day. See the chart above for suggestions for themes and occasions for planning your health fair.

Targeting promotional efforts to specific employee groups also can enhance participation. Groups can be classified by various characteristics such as age, gender, race, specific risk factors, previous participation, and so on. For example, back programs can be directed to workers in labor-intensive jobs; prenatal health education programs for women; exercise programs for clerical personnel; and consumer education and self-care programs for employees who filed a health care claim in the previous year.

To encourage a good turnout with active participation at the fair, consider using plan A or plan B:

PLAN A

1. As they enter the health fair, give each employee a separate "health card."

2. Ask them to read and follow the instructions listed on the card to qualify for a healthy reward (e.g., popcorn, apples, or other healthy snacks) and several grand prizes (e.g., a personal health book, exercise clothing, membership to a health club).

3. Ask each exhibitor/vendor to mark the employee's card after they *participate* in the activity. This will deter employees from merely walking to each station just to get their card marked.

PLAN B

1. Have each vendor type several questions pertaining to their exhibit and display them on a stand-up display card at their table.

2. Make an answer sheet with True and False columns corresponding to each question. Give employees one answer sheet per exhibit and instruct them to write their name and department on each sheet.

3. Encourage employees to complete an answer sheet at each exhibit and to hand it to the exhibitor, who will check it for right and wrong answers (exhibitors should point out any incorrect answers and correct them with the employee). When the answer sheet is totally correct, employees can place it in a "drop bag" to enter random drawings for prizes donated by the exhibitors.

What Would You Do?

After reading the four case studies below, choose one to which you will apply the strategies described in this chapter relevant to the following four components.

1. Customer research (how will you identify employee needs and interests?)

2. Marketing (create a marketing mix)

3. Development and implementation (describe how you will develop and implement your program)

4. Evaluation (describe what variables you will measure to determine programmatic impact)

Case Study #1: A coal mine in New Mexico employs 85 percent Navajo American Indians. Total employee population is 375 people (90 percent men and 10 percent women). Employees are unionized and work three rotating 8-hour shifts. The mine has three sites with separate entrances. The union participates in a nationwide health plan negotiated specifically for coal miners; the plan includes little preventive care. Management will only participate and pay for health promotion activities if employees drive the program.

Case Study #2: A refinery in the Gulf Coast area employs 90 percent men and 10 percent women. The total employee population is 1,200, with an average age of 42. The non-union plant requires 70 percent blue-collar work and works two rotating 12-hour shifts. A health promotion program has been in place for 2 years with an on-site facility of 10,000 square feet. The top employee risk factors are poor eating habits, stress, back injuries, high blood cholesterol, and lack of exercise.

Case Study #3: In a large midwestern city, a cellular phone company has five worksites with 1,500 white-collar employees. The population is 50 percent male and 50 percent female, with an average age of 34. The majority of employees have a college education and the company is non-union. Access to health promotion and risk-reduction programs is limited to the choice of two managed care programs.

Case Study #4: Located on the east coast are 55 offshore oil platforms that house 15 to 40 employees at each bunkhouse. Each facility has a catered food arrangement and 17 have functioning fitness facilities. The population is non-union and 90 percent blue-collar males. The employees belong to a traditional indemnity (fee-for-service) plan, and emergency care is the most common claim.

5

EVALUATING HEALTH
PROMOTION EFFORTS

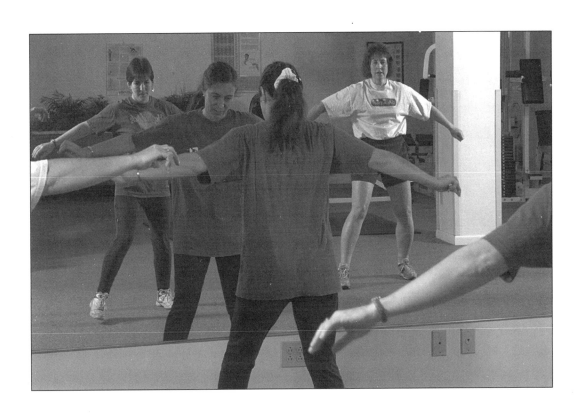

Once a program is underway, program planners should anticipate that management will want to know whether the program is making a positive impact. The evaluation process should have been set up, at least in part, during the planning phase (see chapter 3). In this chapter we'll present rationale for program evaluation and discuss factors program planners must take into account when conducting program evaluations.

EVALUATION PLAN

Several decades ago, Edward Suchman, one of America's great social researchers, said this about program evaluation:

All social institutions or subsystems, whether medical, educational, religious, economic, or political, are required to provide proof of their legitimacy and effectiveness in order to justify society's continued support. Both the demand for and the type of acceptable proof will depend largely on the nature of the relationship between the social institution and the public. In general, a balance will be struck between faith and fact, reflecting the degree of man's respect for authority and tradition within the particular system versus his skepticism and desire for tangible proof of work.

Perhaps Suchman meant to remind us that any intervention (x-rays, a fitness program, health risk appraisal, etc.) needs substantiation. Since Suchman's day, research methods have vastly improved, allowing for more objectivity and a higher degree of validity. It is now inexcusable to base evaluation efforts on assumptions or inappropriate criteria. Rather, the evaluation process should follow standard procedures that have been refined over years (see figure 5.1).

These questions should be addressed before evaluation begins:

- What information should we get from an evaluation?
- What information cannot be obtained through evaluation?
- Do we know how to properly evaluate a program? Do we have the resources we need?
- What criteria should we use to develop an appropriate evaluation?
- When is the best time to conduct an evaluation?
- How do we use evaluation results to help employees and management?

- Should we conduct a comprehensive evaluation or focus on one or two aspects of a program?
- Which program goals are valued most highly by management?
- Which goals are of greatest interest to employees?

DECIDING WHAT TO EVALUATE: GOALS AND OBJECTIVES

Evaluation ties in closely with program goals (see Setting Appropriate Goals in chapter 3, p. 34). Once program goals have been established, evaluating the program is relatively easy. However, because of the time and expense involved in WHP programs, the evaluation process must usually begin before the results are in. After a 4-month program that has cost thousands of dollars, management does not want to hear that none of the goals were met. Thus, program planners must evaluate the program while it's going on (**process evaluation**), especially when a program's goals are long-term. For example, suppose that a goal for a low back injury prevention program is to reduce the number of workers' compensation claims caused by back injuries. How would you evaluate, *during the program,* if this goal is likely to be achieved? One way is by looking at the **program objectives** that have been set toward meeting the long-term goal. For our purposes, objectives can be defined as narrow, measurable checkpoints on the way toward reaching a long-term goal. To be most valuable for the program planner, objectives should be

- tangible or visible,
- measurable,
- relevant to the goal, and
- implemented within a designated timeframe.

QUESTIONS ADDRESSED BY EVALUATION

WHP personnel should expect these questions and know how to answer them:
- Does a health promotion program influence a company's bottom line?
- Do all participants benefit from such a program?
- Can these programs really cut absenteeism, turnover, and health care utilization and boost productivity?
- What type of program is most cost-effective?
- How long does it take for a program to break even?

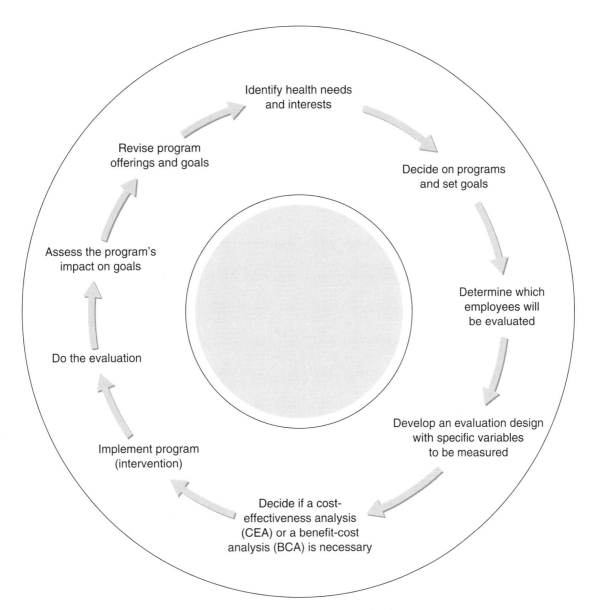

Figure 5.1 Procedural steps in planning and conducting a program evaluation.

DECIDING WHEN TO EVALUATE

Before setting an evaluation time frame, worksite personnel should consider their resources and evaluation capabilities, employees' work schedules, program times, record-keeping systems, and overall costs involved. For example, what percentage of employees have a flextime work schedule rather than a standard work shift? Can an observation be done more efficiently by measuring employees individually, in small groups, or in a large group?

USING A TIME FRAME

Structuring objectives within a time frame will help evaluators periodically monitor each objective. For example, a *long-term objective* might be to reduce absenteeism among hypertensive employees to no more than a 5 percent annual increase over the next 5 years (see figure 5.2) An *intermediate objective* could be to determine if all diagnosed hypertensive employees have successfully entered a risk-reduction program within 2 months of being identified (see figure 5.3). Finally, a *short-term objective* might be to identify at least 5 more hypertensive employees each month and 60 by year-end (see figure 5.4).

EVALUATION DECISIONS

Following are some basic decisions the program planner will need to make during program evaluation.

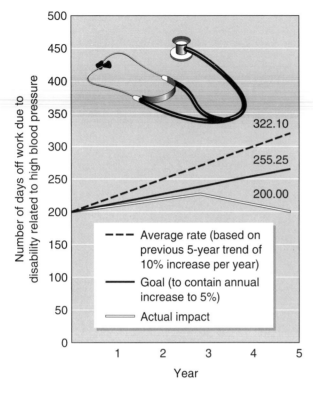

Figure 5.2 Actual and projected absences due to hypertension-related conditions.

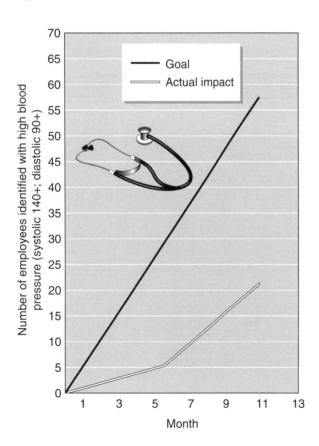

Figure 5.3 Number of employees identified with hypertension at monthly intervals.

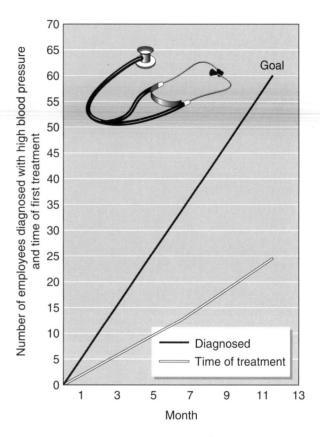

Figure 5.4 A graphic illustration of the number of hypertensive employees at time of diagnosis and time of first treatment.

All of these questions should be answered before the first steps are taken toward evaluation.

• What is the most appropriate measurement tool to use in an observation? Should you use questionnaires, an HRA, physical measurements, or some other tool? Remember that measurement tools should meet two minimum criteria:

1. Each tool should accurately measure what it is supposed to measure. That is, the tool needs to have a high level of validity.

2. Each tool should reliably produce consistent results on repeated observations.

• How many observations should be done? Participants usually prefer regular feedback, whereas management may request only baseline and outcome measurements. In some situations, you may need to strike a compromise.

• What evaluation design should be used? Many designs exist, but only a few are practical for worksite settings.

SHORT-TERM OBJECTIVES

Short-term objectives may include various intervention strategies phased in over time, such as over a year. A code using the letters A through D has been established at many worksites to distinguish types of interventions. These interventions are presented here as they would be introduced over a 1-year low back injury prevention program.

A. Identification. Identify all employees at high risk of back injuries by assessing employees' health histories, workers' compensation records, and on-site injury data (January).

B. Incentive. Offer an incentive for high-risk employees to attend a program orientation (February).

C. Awareness and motivation. Provide weekly awareness activities to motivate employees to practice on-the-job healthy back routines (March-December).

D. Reward. For each month a participant reports no back pain or injury, he can deposit a "lottery ticket" to become eligible for a major prize in the end-of-the-year sweepstakes (March–December).

EVALUATION DESIGN

An evaluation design includes the following essential components (see figure 5.5):

- Observation (O): This is when a measurement is performed.

- Independent variable (X): The program or strategy designed to produce a positive outcome.

- Experimental group (E). The group of employees that participates in the program or strategy.

- Control group (C). The group of nonparticipating employees being compared to the experimental group.

As evaluation designs vary significantly in their scope and specificity, you'll need to tailor your design to the specific needs and interests of your worksite. Several examples of program evaluation design follow.

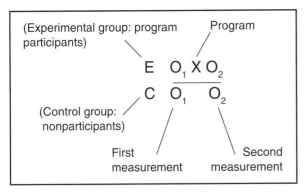

Figure 5.5 Major parts of a sample evaluation design.

ONE GROUP, PRETEST AND POST-TEST

Perhaps the most basic design is the "one group, pretest and post-test design" illustrated in figure 5.6. This design consists of a single measurement before a program is implemented and a second evaluation at the conclusion of the program. This design is easy to conduct in worksite settings but has two major limitations:

1. Since there are no measurements taken during the program, evaluators have to wait until the end of the program to determine if the program made an impact.

2. Since there's no control group, an extraneous variable—weather, change in company policy, change in work responsibilities, change in personal health status, and so on—could influence the outcome. Beautiful weather, for example, might move participants in a worksite weight-management program to exercise outside the program. They may play sports, swim, bike, or go on family hikes. Without a control group (which may also be likely to exercise in good weather), it is difficult to measure the direct impact of the weight-management intervention, as it was supplemented with at-home exercise.

Despite the drawbacks to this design, it remains a popular choice at smaller worksites and for program directors with very limited resources.

PRETEST AND POST-TEST WITH A CONTROL GROUP

Using a control group for comparison always yields more reliable results (see figure 5.7). Presumably

	Pre-program measurement	Program	Post-program measurement
	O_1	X	O_2

Figure 5.6 A one-group pretest and post-test design.

the control group and the experimental group would have exercised the same amount outside of work, on average, and so would have experienced equal or similar benefits from their at-home exercise. Thus, the difference between the two groups in the amount of weight lost would be attributed to the worksite weight-management program (see figure 5.7). Only by comparing the two groups can the evaluators measure the direct impact of the weight-management program.

	Pre-program measurement	Program	Post-program measurement
(E) Participants	O_1	X	O_2
(C) Nonparticipants	O_1		O_2

Figure 5.7 A pretest–post-test control group design.

MULTIPLE-TIME SERIES DESIGN

One of the most respected designs applied in worksite settings is the multiple-time series (MTS) design, as shown in figure 5.8. This design is especially suited for evaluators who have access to past (retrospective) and future (prospective) data or who can conduct measurements on a regular basis.

Suppose a company has established a voluntary back stretching program to reduce the prevalence and cost of back injuries. Different types of MTS designs can be used to evaluate the program, as-

	Pre-program measurements	Program begins	Program measurements
E (participants)	O_1 O_2 O_3	X	O_4 O_5 O_6
C (nonparticipants)	O_1 O_2 O_3		O_4 O_5 O_6
	Jan. Mar. May	July	Aug. Oct. Dec.

Figure 5.8 A sample multiple-time series design.

suming evaluators can measure the number of low back injuries that occurred before, during, and after the program.

Measurements are taken before the program to determine if one group is noticeably different from the other group. By comparing any change in the number of back injuries among participants (O_1 to O_2) with any change in the number of back injuries among nonparticipants (O_1 to O_2), evaluators can compare injury rates between the two groups prior to the program. In addition, injury data for both groups can be compared a second time (O_2 to O_3) to give evaluators greater insight about any pre-program differences that may exist between the groups. If one group shows significantly fewer back injuries than the other group prior to the program, evaluators could select a different group of nonparticipants for comparison. Ideally, this comparison group would have a similar number of back injuries to the participant group. If not, then a third group of nonparticipants could be chosen and so on, until a comparison group similar to the experimental group was identified.

Since random assignment is not required in MTS designs, it's possible for participants to be inherently different from nonparticipants. For example, suppose a company suspects that a high percentage of employees is using a local hospital's emergency department for minor, nonemergency health problems. A review of health care claims shows 75 percent of suspected emergency department abuses were incurred by employees under 40 years of age. While in the process of planning a new medical self-care program to minimize this problem, the company distributed surveys on three pre-program occasions (O_1, O_2, and O_3) to assess employee interest in a self-care program. Suppose employees who expressed the highest interest in the program on the first occasion (O_1) also reported the most visits to the emergency department over the past year. Yet, on the second (O_2) and third (O_3) occasions, responding employees reportedly had the lowest rate of emergency department visits. By assessing employee interest on three separate occasions before implementing a self-care program, worksite health personnel were able to see that employees interested in the self-care program actually represented a broad cross-section of employees. They could then use this information to determine if a self-care program should be offered to the entire workforce or directed primarily toward employees under 40.

To minimize the possibility of significant pre-program differences, evaluators should try to match participants and nonparticipants as closely as possible, especially on attributes associated with the outcome variable being measured. For example, studies suggest that an employee's risk of back injury is influenced by the following variables:

Age	Exercise habits
Body weight	Job rotation
History of back injury	Lifting habits
Pre-work stretching	Hamstring and low back
Abdominal strength	flexibility
Work satisfaction	Coping skills (stress)
Type of job	

An effective matching technique is to randomly select nonparticipating employees to form a control group of members who resemble participants. For example, if a new back injury prevention program is being implemented, consider matching the groups on as many criteria as possible related to back injury risk. Since it's unlikely that you can choose nonparticipants who will identically match participants on all relevant criteria, a control group can be qualified if it has some overall resemblance to participants. It's usually necessary to establish an acceptable range for specific criteria. The table below is an example.

Another way to help equate groups is to randomly assign participants to different versions of a program. Random assignment is feasible when a new program has been added to an existing program or when a new program has two or more versions offered simultaneously. Say, for example, you have 50 employees sign up for a smoking-cessation program. You could randomly divide the volunteers into two subgroups of 25 each, then show one group a self-help video and ask the other group to attend on-site seminars (see figure 5.9). Since the groups are selected from one pool of volunteers, there's less chance that one group is inherently different from the other group. This design also allows evaluators to compare one particular intervention with another intervention to determine which is most cost-effective.

$$R \ E_1 \text{ (self-help video)} \quad O_1 \ O_2 \ O_3 \ X \ O_4 \ O_5 \ O_6$$
$$R \ E_2 \text{ (on-site seminars)} \quad O_1 \ O_2 \ O_3 \ X \ O_4 \ O_5 \ O_6$$

Figure 5.9 A sample multiple-time series design with two randomly assigned groups of participants.

ECONOMIC-BASED EVALUATIONS

Management will always want to know which WHP strategies produce the best results for the least expense. Two of the most common economic-based evaluations used in various worksites are **benefit-cost analysis** (BCA) and **cost-effectiveness analysis** (CEA).

	Participants	Nonparticipants in acceptable ranges
Work location	Warehouse	Warehouse
Average age	37 years old	35-40 years old
Average body weight	185 pounds.	175-195 pounds
Past back injuries	1.5 per person	1-2
Exercise habits	Walks a mile a day	Walks .5 to 1.5 miles a day
Rotate jobs	80% do not	70 to 90% do not
Pre-work stretch	90% do not	>80% do not
Lifting habits	15 lifts a day	0-20 lifts a day
Abdominal strength	20 sit-ups in a minute	>15 sit-ups in a minute
Work satisfaction	75% satisfied	> 65% satisfied
High stress level	50%	> 40%

BENEFIT-COST ANALYSIS

The primary purpose of a BCA is to determine whether a program is worth its cost. As the BCA method compares program costs to program benefits, it might be most effective when both benefits and costs can be measured in monetary terms. However, some researchers caution that quantification shouldn't be the sole basis for performing a benefit-cost analysis, contending that important factors should not be neglected just because they cannot be tangibly measured. For example, how would we quantify the suffering of people with severe back pain or chronic depression? Benefit-cost analysis doesn't purport to introduce rigor and quantification when the data are imprecise or where quantification is not feasible. However, when costs and benefits *can* be quantified, a BCA is a simple and handy way to evaluate a program's success or value. For example, suppose a hypertension screening program yields cost-savings of $50,000 in reduced hypertension-related absenteeism and health care expenses. Compare this sum to the program's annual operating cost of $20,000, and you get a 5:2 ratio ($50,000 to $20,000) of benefit to cost.

BCA can also be used to compare two or more programs to see which is most cost-effective. Suppose the hypertension program's benefit-cost ratio is compared to that of a back stretching program with a BC ratio of $20,000 to $3,000 (or $6.66 to $1). Although both programs are successful, the back stretching program produced a better benefit-to-cost ratio.

Let's try doing a BCA on an exercise program implemented at an actual worksite. The major reason for using a BCA was to determine if the exercise program could reduce sick-leave absences among participants. Table 5.1 shows the number of work days missed by participants at two different times: the year prior to the program and the year during the program.

Due to the drop in absenteeism, company costs related to missed work days dropped nearly 70 percent (from $1,046.87 to $703.12). This savings is the "benefit." The company could save nearly $1,500 annually if the program continued without interruption and maintained the initial drop in absenteeism (see table 5.2).

The cost involved in administering this program was considerably lower than the company's cost for absenteeism (see table 5.2).

As shown in table 5.3, benefit dollars from reduced absenteeism exceeded cost dollars by a ratio of nearly 20 to 1. Thus, the program generated sufficient benefits to merit a favorable response and endorsement from management. Note that the preceding results are not typically found in most WHP programs. Nonetheless, programs that generate a marginal benefit-to-cost ratio—even as small as 1%—have produced more than what they cost and, thus, deserve support consideration from all decision makers.

COST-EFFECTIVENESS ANALYSIS

What if program planners want to compare one program with another program to learn which one produces the greatest benefit for the least expense? Properly implemented, cost-effectiveness analysis

---

Table 5.1 A Comparison of Absenteeism Costs One Year Before and One Year During a Worksite Exercise Program

	Before	During
Company's cost per employee (at $12.50 an hour for a 1-day absence)*	$ 100.00	$ 100.00
Number of days off work	183.75	56.25
Total company cost for absenteeism	18,375.00	5,625.00
Difference (savings) = $12,750		

*Based on wages and salaries (including fringe benefits and payroll taxes) averaging $20,000 per employee with an assumed 25 percent return on payroll dollars (not including the cost of temporary replacements). A 25 percent return is based on the amount of money a company expects to use for essential research and development purposes (also called "opportunity costs").

Table 5.2	Costs Related to a Worksite Exercise Program
Area-item	**Cost**
Personnel:	
Registered nurse	$625.00[1]
Consultant	0.00[2]
Exercise leader	0.00[2]
Facility:	
Physical area	Fixed cost[3]
Carpeting (in/outdoor)	Fixed cost[3]
Utilities:	
Lighting	0.00[4]
Heating/cooling	0.00[5]
Equipment:	
Blood pressure kit	0.00[6]
Fat calipers	0.00[6]
Weight scale	0.00[6]
Tape measure	0.00[6]
Flexibility box	0.00[6]
Steps, stool, or chair for step-test	0.00[6]
Cassette player	0.00[6]
Cassette tapes (3)	3.00
Paper products and duplicating	10.00
Total	**$638.00**

[1] Based on the average annual salary of $25,000 for an occupational health nurse in eastern North Carolina; multiplied by .025 (50 hours is annual workload for this program).

[2] Services provided on a voluntary, complimentary basis; the nurse and exercise leader were full-time employees.

[3] Based on the decision, if necessary, to furnish the activity area with indoor-outdoor carpeting at $8.95 per yard for 516.66 yards (4,650 square feet) and replaced once every 10 years.

[4] No cost involved since the exercise area was located where natural daylight provided a sufficient light source.

[5] Heating or cooling expenses were unnecessary due to the moderate climate conditions during the initial 12 weeks of the program (late spring to early summer).

[6] Owned by the company's medical department and provided at no cost.

Table 5.3	Benefit-Cost Comparisons		
	Absolute dollars	**Dollars ratio**	**Net return per investment**
Benefit	$12,750	$19.98	$18.98
Cost	$ 638	$ 1.00	

wanted to know which smoking cessation program is the most cost effective, the CEA framework shown in table 5.4, on the next page, could be implemented.

The data in table 5.4 suggest that the "cold turkey" program was less costly to provide at this worksite and three times more economical (one-third as costly) as the gradual withdrawal approach.

CONDUCTING A COST-EFFECTIVENESS ANALYSIS

Conducting a CEA in a worksite setting involves several key steps:

1. Determining the program's objectives. What, specifically, is the program designed to do for the employees and the company?

2. Determining the total operating costs. Consider both major cost items (personnel, facilities, equipment) and minor cost items (photocopying, record keeping). (You might need help from your company accountant during this phase.)

3. Determining the outcome of each program used to meet a desired goal. Compare the outcomes of all strategies.

4. Compare program outcomes and determine which is most cost-effective (see table 5.5). Although the seminar/belt intervention program initially cost five times as much as the daily stretch intervention, the stretch routine produced a higher return on investment. The stretch protected employees against a back injury at nearly one-seventh ($20 vs. $135) the cost of the seminar/belt combination.

Although a CEA may show one program having a greater **return on investment** than another program, the decision to eliminate a particular program should not be based solely on this comparison alone.

(CEA) can answer that question. Rather than assigning monetary values to a single outcome of a program, as is done in benefit-cost analysis, CEA compares only the costs of similar programs for achieving a specific outcome. For example, if you

Table 5.4 A Cost-Effectiveness Analysis Framework Used in Comparing Two Different Smoking-Cessation Interventions

		Participants		Quitters	
Type of program	**Cost of program**	**Number of**	**Cost per**	**Number of**	**Cost* per**
Cold turkey with self-help booklet	$2,000	100	$20	50	$ 40
Gradual withdrawal with on-site counselor	3,000	100	30	25	120

*Cost of program divided by number of quitters.

Table 5.5 A Cost-Effectiveness Analysis of Two Worksite Programs

Program	Cost/year	Procedure/outcome	Cost/outcome
Monthly back seminar with lumbar back belt	$5,000	100 screenings	$50 per screen
		50 diagnosed as high risk due to poor back flexibility and/or abdominal weakness	$100 per positive find
		40 participated	$125 per participant
		37 reported no low back injury in first year of program	$135 per positive outcome
Daily pre-work stretching	$1,000	100 screenings	$10 per screen
		80 diagnosed as high risk due to poor back flexibility and/or abdominal weakness	$12.50 per positive find
		75 participated in daily stretching	$13.33 per participant
		50 reported no low back injury within one year of seminar	$20 per positive find

After all, a program with a moderate return on investment may produce benefits that are not easily quantified (e.g., enhanced employee morale and better management-labor relations).

EVALUATING TO PRODUCE INFORMATION

Some evaluators make the mistake of planning an evaluation after a WHP program is under way rather than during the planning phase. In these cases evaluation procedures are often rushed and off base, resulting in unreliable results. Good planning gives evaluators enough time to properly lay out important parameters of an evaluation, such as

- what variables will be measured,
- what employees to target,
- who will conduct the evaluation,
- who should have access to the results,
- how much financial support is needed,
- what equipment and instruments are needed,
- what evaluation procedures are most efficient, and
- how the results are going to be used.

As an evaluator, you should incorporate six basic guidelines in planning and conducting these parameters:

1. Have some idea what you're looking for. Decide what factors and outcomes are most important to track.

2. Try to be in a position where you can act on the results. Secure management support and form alliances with departments handling essential data (personnel, safety, benefits, human resources).

3. Follow sound and normal statistical procedures. For example, does absenteeism need to be distinguished as controllable or uncontrollable? Were previous cost savings adjusted to reflect today's market value?

4. Recognize normal versus abnormal results. A slight drop in absenteeism among program participants may be normal, but a 100 percent quit rate among smokers would be unrealistic.

5. Monitor each variable you're measuring. How many participants are losing body weight at a healthy rate? What types of health care claims are rising the fastest?

6. Try to convert data into valuable information. Focus on evolving trends. What trends are occurring in certain age groups and departments?

What Would You Do?

Upon reviewing HRAs and health care claims data, you notice an increase in diabetes-related cases and costs compared to the previous year's experience. While preparing a proposal for a diabetes education and management program, you anticipate that your boss will ask you how the program will be evaluated and when the program will begin to pay off. What type of evaluation is most appropriate—a benefit-cost analysis or a break-even analysis? Which technique would you choose and why?

WORKSITE

HEALTH PROMOTION

PROGRAMS

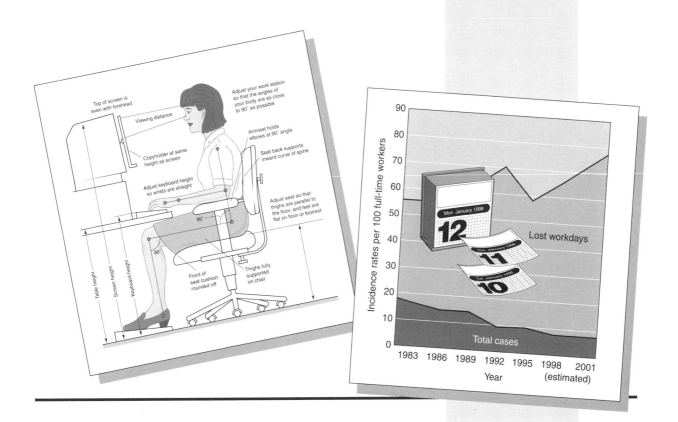

BUILDING A HEALTHY WORK ENVIRONMENT

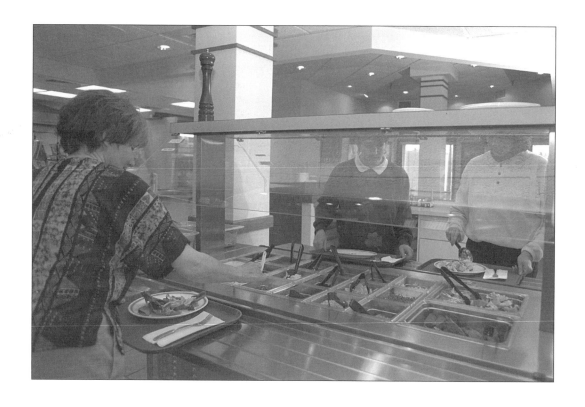

One of the biggest challenges facing employers is reducing major health risks among employees. Much of their success will hinge on the extent to which they can prevent injuries, develop a positive worksite culture in which health is valued, maintain an assistance program for employees to turn to when necessary, and help employees manage the daily stress they encounter at work. In this chapter we will discuss various ways of dealing with the work-related issues of maintaining a successful WHP program.

Developing a Healthy Worksite Culture

A question all employers and WHP program directors need to ask is, *Are the employee habits promoted at our company healthy or unhealthy?* Take three worksites, for example: one permits cigarette smoking anywhere in the worksite, the second restricts smoking to certain areas, and the third bans smoking completely. The cultural norm (i.e., expected behavior) in the first company is that smoking is a perfectly fine thing to do; in the third company the norm is that smoking is not acceptable, at least not at the worksite. Which of these norms would you want to promote at your site?

Instituting Change

It should come as no surprise that employees are more motivated to lead healthy lifestyles in a worksite that places a high priority on health. Company policies that do not promote healthy lifestyles should be reconsidered and changed. In most cases, change should be gradually phased in so employees have time (usually a matter of weeks for a minor change and a matter of months or even years for a major change) to adjust to new policies. For example, Nortel (formerly Northern Telecom) and Pacific Bell phased in a series of worksite smoking restrictions over two years before fully implementing their comprehensive clean air (smoke-free) policies. Positive responses far outnumbered the negative at both worksites. Prior to establishing any major changes in policy, management may take a few months to solicit employees' opinions on the proposed change. Yet, in some instances, management may have decided the change is needed and chooses not to solicit employees' feedback. In both cases, a company will usually spend several months educating employees about the need for the proposed change. Depending on the type of program or policy being proposed, a company may choose to introduce it on a trial basis, say, in certain locations or with a particular group of employees, and then expand it to the remainder of the workforce within a designated timeframe. (See chapter 7 for a step-by-step process to phase in a clean-air policy.)

Strategies for Inspiring Change

Depending on an organization's culture and goals, an employer or WHP program director can implement various health promotion strategies to promote and reinforce healthy behaviors. These strategies might be general or more specific, such as taking an ergonomic approach or emphasizing exercise or education.

Ergonomic Strategies

Ergonomics is a science concerned with the characteristics of people that need to be considered in designing and arranging things so that people and things can interact effectively and safely. In WHP, ergonomics involves designing or placing equipment to be used by employees to make each employee's work tasks more efficient or safe. For example, to minimize musculoskeletal injuries and boost productivity, a worksite might purchase state-of-the-art office equipment (e.g., custom chairs that adjust to suit each employee's needs) that minimizes risk of overuse injuries.

Exercise Strategies

Many employees appreciate the opportunity to exercise as an end in itself, for the pure enjoyment of it. It so happens that while they are enjoying the physical exertion they are also becoming more productive and healthy. Some ideas for initiating exercise strategies at the worksite include

- setting up a free weights area in the fitness center—a popular feature for bodybuilders and competitive weight lifters or others who simply want to tone muscles;

- providing stationary bikes or recumbent bikes in suitable locations throughout the worksite for employees to use during breaks and lunchtime;

- encouraging employees who sit a lot to take a "stretch break" for better circulation and work efficiency;

- equipping a designated break area with basketball goals, table tennis, horseshoe pits, and other recreational equipment; and

- developing trails near the worksite and encouraging employees to walk or jog during breaks and over lunch.

EDUCATION STRATEGIES

Some employers in the appropriate kind of work environment may choose to offer employees the opportunity to educate themselves on health issues during regular work hours. Other companies provide employees with informative materials to take home to read if they choose. While it's more likely that employees will read the material if they are reading during work time rather than their own time, there are many worksites where it's not feasible or practical to encourage employees to read on the job (except during lunchtime or on breaks). Here are some possible ways to make educational material available to employees, though not all of them will be appropriate at every facility:

• Stock a cart with health magazines, books, and brochures and periodically move the cart to different locations throughout the worksite.

• Place health magazine racks in bathroom stalls.

• Include a Personal Health column in the company newsletter.

• Ask influential managers to write regular worksite health program endorsement letters in the company newsletter or subscribe to a monthly health promotion newsletter for employees to read and share with their families.

GENERAL STRATEGIES

Along with specific ergonomic, exercise, and educational strategies, here are some more general tactics that employers might try to promote healthy changes of habit. Some of them are very easy to apply; others will take some time, and you might want to implement them gradually.

• Offer many accessible water fountains and distribute "mailbites" to inform employees of the benefits of hydration and the fact that most people do not drink enough water each day.

• Convert a 10-by-10-foot area into a "Personal Health Satellite," a self-contained screening and resource module equipped with an automatic blood pressure cuff, weight scales, health brochures, and other exhibits.

• Designate a period of time for employees to participate in company-sponsored health promotion activities. For example, devote the first 5 minutes of the work shift to stretching exercises, or add 15 minutes to lunch for employees to attend a "Lunch 'n Learn" seminar or to take a walk.

• Review the company's sick leave policy to determine if "sick days" can be renamed to convey a more positive connotation for employees ("Personal Health Days," for example).

• Offer employees with excellent attendance a financial bonus or an additional "health promotion" day for each day their absenteeism for a period falls under the company average. (*Important note:* Work with Human Resources to ensure that the policy does not discourage employees with real illnesses from seeking necessary health care.)

• Establish smoke-free and safety belt use policies in all company vehicles.

Building a positive, health-minded culture at the worksite cannot be done in a day—or even in a few days or weeks. The development will take some time and is best done gradually. Programs implemented too quickly often vanish as fast as they appear. Gradual change is much more reliable. A WHP director should never spring large new programs on employees all at once. Small, gradual changes can combine to alter a culture's values—big sweeping changes are usually met with resistance.

Along with developing a work culture that values health and fitness, a company must constantly monitor conditions at the worksite to ensure the facility and equipment are as safe as possible in order to prevent injury. Accidents will always occur, but if management responds properly to the mishap, the same accident should never occur twice.

PREVENTING OCCUPATIONAL INJURY

In 1970 the Occupational Safety and Health Act was established to encourage and mandate American employers to provide safe workplaces for their employees. Since then the incidence of occupational illnesses and injuries has decreased nearly 25 percent, yet, as illustrated in figure 6.1, the number of lost workdays has increased nearly 60 percent! Despite the decreased incidence, employers annually report over 6 million occupational injuries and illnesses, with an injury-to-illness ratio of 20 to 1.

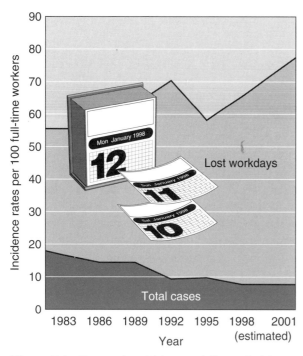

Figure 6.1 Occupational injury and illness incidence rates per 100 full-time workers.

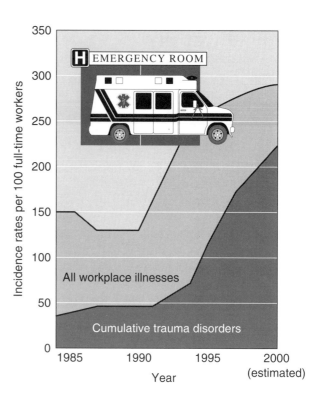

Figure 6.2 Incidence rates for CTDs compared to all workplace illnesses.

Nearly half of all on-the-job ailments lead to serious work restrictions or lost work time. Moreover, the Social Security Administration predicts that over the next 10 years an aging baby-boomer–generation workforce will lead to a 37-percent increase in the incidence of disability. The most common worksite injuries in the United States are **cumulative trauma disorders** (CTDs), such as carpal tunnel syndrome. These injuries occur over time, usually as a result of performing one or more movements repeatedly day after day.

CUMULATIVE TRAUMA DISORDERS

Cumulative trauma disorders affect approximately 18 million U.S. workers annually. About 2 million of these suffer from some degree of carpal tunnel syndrome, 4 million get tendinitis, and about 8.5 million have CTD-related low back pain. Furthermore, since 1980 the incidence of CTDs has risen nearly 600 percent. Recent studies indicate that CTDs have affected about 50 percent of supermarket cashiers, 41 percent of meatpackers, 40 percent of newspaper workers, and 22 percent of telecommunications workers. CTDs now account for more

than half of all workplace illnesses (see figure 6.2), and thus far there is no indication that this percentage will decrease in the near future. In fact, studies show that about 75 percent of *all* American workers will experience a CTD back injury sometime during their working lives. See the section on back health in chapter 7 (pp. 94-96) for more information on CTD back injuries.

THE CAUSES OF CTDS

What causes CTDs? Many factors may contribute to an employee being afflicted with a CTD, including poorly designed equipment, fast-paced work, few or no rest breaks, stress, poor posture, force and repetition, individual predisposition, and poor physical condition. Research suggests that employers are becoming more aware of the costliness of CTDs, which should lead to more care taken in the purchase of supplies. However, the expense of specially made equipment to reduce CTDs prevents many companies from buying them. As more attention is given to the huge costs of CTDs, there will be even greater demand for specialized equipment, and the prices should start to come down.

STUDIES ON CTD PREVENTION STRATEGIES

Many studies indicate a positive relationship between reduced injury and specific programs. For example, a study by Canadian researchers investigated the impact of a physical fitness program on job-related injuries and associated costs at a municipal worksite. Each of the 134 participants was tested for back fitness, strength, aerobic power, flexibility, weight, body fat percentage, blood pressure, lifestyle, and productivity. Participants were given an exercise prescription based on their overall fitness level. After 6 months of exercising, participants were retested and exhibited a 14.2-percent increase in their overall back fitness level. Moreover, injury-related absences dropped one fourth of a day (while nonparticipants' absences increased approximately 3.1 days), producing an estimated cost-savings of $62,922.

These results resemble those of an investigation to determine the effect of physical fitness upon back injuries in fire fighters. To ensure high fitness levels, the program provided each participant with 3 hours of exercise per week and periodically assessed him or her for the duration of the study. Overall, the study indicated that physical fitness and conditioning prevented back injuries. Moreover, the study showed a statistically significant drop in the number of injuries sustained with a corresponding gain in physical fitness. A follow-up study spanned 14 years and showed that enhanced fitness levels strongly corresponded to lower injury rates and associated costs. The fittest employees had only one-eighth as many injuries as the least fit employees, and unfit workers incurred twice as many low back injury costs as fit workers. In addition, workers' compensation claims dropped by half for the entire department over the last 8 years of the study, and disability costs declined 25 percent. (It should be noted that these improvements are probably the result of both the physical fitness program and changes in the administration of the return-to-work program.)

One researcher studied the effect of two 5-minute exercise breaks on musculoskeletal strain among data-entry operators. The exercises were designed to relieve cervicobrachial posture strain but also included the arm, wrist, and lower leg manipulation. In the 2 years before the introduction of the exercise program there were, at any one time, 7 to 12 active CTD-based workers' compensation claims on behalf of injured operators. In the year following the introduction of the program, there were no new claims. There was also an immediate 25 percent climb in productivity and a cost savings in overtime reported in other areas.

RESEARCH CONCLUSIONS

Most of the research published from the 1980s to the present indicates that WHP reduces the incidence, severity, and associated costs of CTDs. Studies also indicate that regular exercisers have no greater risk of sustaining musculoskeletal injuries than non-exercisers and occasional exercisers. Nevertheless, most of the CTD-based studies focus primarily on back injuries and do not address other CTDs such as carpal tunnel syndrome and other repetitive motion injuries.

Studies on the potential influence of WHP on CTDs generate several yet unanswered questions:

1. What types of personal factors actually influence injury risk?

2. Are these factors as influential at all types of worksites or only in specific types of worksite?

3. Can specific factors be influenced by voluntary lifestyle changes resulting from a WHP intervention?

4. Which intervention makes the greatest impact for the least cost?

5. If WHP interventions carry great potential for success with CTDs, are American employers prepared to implement them?

Some health care professionals suggest that workers who regularly engage in vigorous, "whole body" exercise such as swimming or jogging have a much lower risk for carpal tunnel syndrome and possibly other types of CTDs. See chapter 7 for more discussion of physical fitness programs. Here, we will look at other interventions that can help prevent or deal with cumulative trauma disorders.

STRATEGIES FOR CTD PREVENTION

The strategies health experts recommend to employers for reducing the risk of CTDs at the workplace include adjusting work stations to fit individual

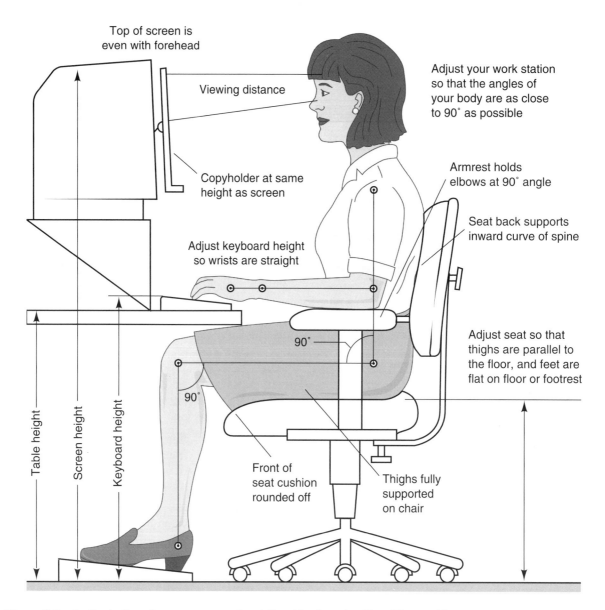

Top of screen is
even with forehead

Viewing distance

Adjust your work station
so that the angles of
your body are as close
to 90° as possible

Copyholder at same
height as screen

Armrest holds
elbows at 90° angle

Seat back supports
inward curve of spine

Adjust keyboard height
so wrists are straight

90°

Adjust seat so that
thighs are parallel to
the floor, and feet are
flat on floor or footrest

Table height

Screen height

Keyboard height

90°

Front of
seat cushion
rounded off

Thighs fully
supported
on chair

Figure 6.3   An illustration of proper ergonomic relationships for a healthy sitting position.

needs (see figure 6.3); providing indirect light to minimize glare; providing adjustable chairs with armrests and good low back support; and supplying video display terminals with antiglare hoods, tiltable screens, and resting pads for hands and wrists. These basic strategies can be expensive but are relatively easy to implement and will significantly reduce CTDs. Strategies that are less easy to initiate—because they involve more than just purchasing new equipment—but which are less expensive and could prove just as beneficial in the long run involve conducting education and training sessions, encouraging employees to take more breaks, and monitoring employees to make sure their work practices are not endangering them for CTDs.

EMPLOYEE ASSISTANCE PROGRAMS

Considering the stresses of balancing home and worklife demands, quality of worklife initiatives are making inroads in the workplace. According to several surveys, more employers are recognizing that employees need flexible human resource and benefit programs throughout their working years to help them deal with various health-related changes. For example, more employers are offering **life cycle benefit** programs that include aspects of health promotion and fitness incentives for employees and

Table 6.1 Sample Components in a Life Cycle Benefits Program		
Covered expense	**You will be reimbursed**	**Annual maximum**
• Housing assistance	After 4 years of service, for the purchase of a primary residence only	$1,000
• Healthy lifestyle	For a health club membership, quitting smoking, losing weight, etc.	400
• Financial planning	For financial planning by a qualified financial planner or the purchase of computer-based financial planning software	250
• Childcare, eldercare	For the services of a nonfamily childcare/eldercare provider; for an adoption referral service	300
• Legal assistance	For legal assistance in connection with wills, estates, and adoption	200

dependents. These benefit programs allow employees to tailor their benefits package according to whatever their greatest needs are at the time. Employees can choose from a varied menu of benefits offerings, including those listed in table 6.1.

Many life cycle benefit programs have evolved from programs called **employee assistance programs,** or EAPs. Currently more than 10,000 American employers provide EAPs, compared to only 50 in the early 1970s. Although the original EAPs—established in the early 1950s—were designed primarily to help alcoholic workers and dependents, most of today's EAPs provide a full spectrum of services including financial counseling, substance abuse treatment, elder care, child care, and retirement planning. The most common problems reported through EAPs today concern emotional, job-related, and personal relationship problems (see figure 6.4).

ADMINISTRATIVE ISSUES

Developing and operating effective life cycle benefit and EAP programs involve various administrative issues. Among the most important issues are administrative positioning, staffing, services, sites, and participation criteria.

POSITIONING

Integrating an EAP within a comprehensive health promotion framework is becoming more popular because doing so

- maximizes resources, especially for smaller companies with limited finances,

- makes the working environment healthier as more people work toward a common goal,

- reduces the stigma associated with getting personal help—as part of a comprehensive program, workers are more likely to view EAP services in the same way as other health promotion programs, and

- helps meet the total needs of high-risk workers as programs can be tailored to help individuals with psychological problems related to alcoholism, anorexia nervosa, recent heart attacks, and other personal health crises.

However, there are also potential drawbacks to an integrated approach. These include the possibility that sharing resources may limit allocations and jeopardize the potential impact of an EAP; that EAP services may be underrepresented if another health promotion component (the fitness center, for example) becomes too visible; that employees may underestimate the importance of an EAP and not seek help; and that other health promotion programs may inadvertently try to address EAP-related issues. It is important that other programs complement EAP services rather than trying to replace them.

STAFFING

Not just anyone should volunteer to be a member of the EAP staff. Due to the complex issues involved in dealing with the problems typically referred to EAP personnel, staffing guidelines should be followed as closely as possible. First of all, staff members should be professionally trained and certified in the areas of mental health and substance abuse.

Referrals By Problem Type

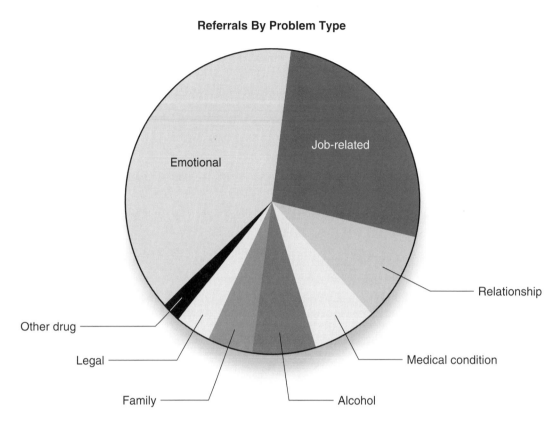

Figure 6.4   The most common problems reported to a randomly selected group of EAPs.

Each staff member should be evaluated once a year. Managers and union representatives should be kept informed of any EAP staffing changes and how these changes affect responsibilities. To minimize the chance of malpractice and liability claims, employers should conduct a legal review of the EAP and keep thorough files of all EAP activity. Finally, the overall impact of the program should be evaluated by an outside firm every 2 to 4 years.

ESTABLISHING AN EAP SITE

Each on-site and off-site EAP has its own advantages and drawbacks. An on-site EAP may give a company greater opportunity to perform quality control measures, but workers may wonder if their identities can be protected. In contrast, some workers may find it either inconvenient or indiscreet to visit an off-site EAP. Whether an on-site or off-site EAP would suit your situation better may also depend on financial considerations. Larger employers are usually more likely to staff and fund an in-house EAP. However, many companies, large and small, opt to use an alternative arrangement, such

as an off-site consortium or an internal referral system.

CONSORTIUM

In a typical consortium arrangement a group of employers pay a local EAP organization—for example, the mental health center—to provide services to employees and their dependents. Usually the fee for these services will depend on the size of workforce. For example, if an employer has a workforce of 100 employees, the employer may pay $5 for each employee ($500) plus a base rate of $1,000, for a total cost of $1,500 a year. Employers with a larger group of employees may pay the same per-employee rate of $5 but a much higher base rate.

INTERNAL REFERRAL

In this arrangement supervisors trained in EAP issues identify employees with personal problems that may be affecting their attendance, productivity, or morale. The troubled employees may be referred to an on-site EAP coordinator or to a designated EAP provider in the community for counseling. A common referral process is shown in figure 6.5.

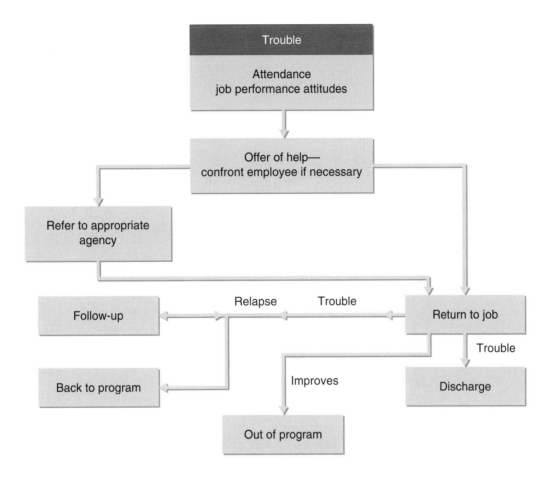

Figure 6.5 An internal referral EAP framework.

SUBSTANCE ABUSE PREVENTION AND TREATMENT

A common goal of life cycle and EAP programs is to prevent and treat substance abuse. Historically, substance abuse prevention and treatment strategies centered on alcohol, but today prescription medication abuse and illegal drug use are also emphasized.

THE SCOPE OF THE PROBLEM

Substance abuse has a formidable economic impact on businesses. Consider these statistics:

- Lost productivity and quality defects related to substance abuse cost American businesses over $45 billion each year.

- Each substance abuser costs his or her employer over $7,500 a year in lost productivity, increased medical care, and damaged property.

- At least 10 percent of America's health care costs is due to substance abuse.

- Approximately 10 percent of American workers abuse alcohol and/or other drugs.

- Nearly 50 percent of all industrial accidents involve alcohol.

- Forty percent of all worksite deaths are traced to alcohol abuse.

The National Institute on Drug Abuse (NIDA) estimated the incidence of illegal drug and heavy alcohol use among workers in specific industries and found the following:

	Percentage of workers	
Industry	**Use illegal drugs**	**Drink heavily**
Construction	21.6	17.0
Repair services	18.5	6.5
Wholesale trade	15.9	2.3
Professional	11.3	2.9
Retail trade	11.2	10.1
Manufacturing	10.3	3.3
Finance	9.3	3.8

Here are some strategies employers use in dealing with substance abuse:

• Publicize a written statement on the costs and health risks associated with substance abuse and other problems covered by the EAP. This document should be signed by the chief executive and also union representatives when appropriate. The statement should reflect management and labor philosophies and agreements that coincide with EAP objectives.

• Develop written guidelines that specify how records will be maintained, for how long, who will have access to them, what information will be released to whom and under what conditions, and what use, if any, can be made of records for purposes of research, evaluation, and reports.

• Write procedures to inform employees what actions management and union representatives will take at each phase of the program.

• Include diagnosis, treatment, and rehabilitation coverage in the medical/disability benefits plan.

• Operate the EAP within the standards and practices established by one or more of the following associations:

1. Association of Labor-Management Administrators and Consultants on Alcoholism (ALMACA)

2. Employee Assistance Professional Association (EAPA)

3. Employee Assistance Society of North America (EASNA)

4. National Institute on Alcohol Abuse and Alcoholism (NIAAA)

5. National Council on Alcoholism (NCA)

DRUG TESTING

When a company decides to drug test it is wisest to set employee protection and quality preservation as goals for the program. Sound and ethical procedures need to be established to protect employees' rights and minimize litigation. Hire laboratories certified by the College of American Pathologists or the National Institute on Drug Abuse to do the testing. To maximize accuracy, if a urine sample tests positive for drug use the sample should then undergo either radioimmunoassay, gas chromatography, or,

RECOVERY RATES FOR SUBSTANCE ABUSERS

Recovery rates for substance abusers entering treatment through worksite interventions are the highest of any referral source; approximately 60 percent to 80 percent are successfully rehabilitated. Many companies using the most advanced techniques to identify, counsel, and treat troubled individuals are reporting favorable results from their EAP investments. The following examples have been cited by the National Council on Alcoholism:

• **Allis-Chalmers.** Absenteeism dropped from 8 percent to 3 percent and the discharge rate from 95 percent to 8 percent (among participants), producing an estimated savings of $80,000.

• **Consolidated Edison.** Nearly 60 percent of EAP patients are rehabilitated, and absenteeism dropped from 14 days to 4 days per year per patient.

• **Detroit Edison.** Absenteeism dropped 75 percent.

• **Du Pont.** Approximately 66 percent of employee alcoholics have been successfully rehabilitated.

• **Firestone Tire and Rubber.** Accident and sickness costs cut 65 percent.

• **General Motors.** Lost work time cut 40 percent; sickness and accident claims costs down 60 percent; grievance proceedings and job accidents down 50 percent.

• **Illinois Bell.** On-the-job disabling injuries dropped 81 percent.

• **3M Company.** Nearly 80 percent of employee alcoholics either recovered or controlled to the point where noticeable improvements in attendance, productivity, and family and community relationships are evident.

• **McDonnell Douglas.** Estimated $5.1 million savings (reduced health care claims and lower absenteeism) over 3 years.

See appendix A for EAP resources and other topic-specific resources.

preferably, GC/mass spectrometry. These advanced tests (which cost between $40 and $50) break drugs into single molecules and thus confirm or contradict the presence of even small amounts of a particular drug.

Stress Management

According to many employee-based surveys, on-the-job stress is the most common risk factor in today's worksites. Yet, only one of every five worksites provides employee stress-management programs.

The Effects of Stress

Why is worksite stress a problem for employees and employers? Distressed employees have higher rates of absences, accidents, illnesses, and productivity errors than their less-stressed counterparts. Stressed employees also file the majority of stress-related workers' compensation claims, which are climbing to an all-time high.

Programming Tips

Some employers have responded by integrating stress-management counseling services into their EAPs. Additional ways to monitor and reduce employee stress include reviewing health care claims data to determine if stress is in fact a problem at the worksite; converting an unused employee lounge into a quiet, dimly lighted room where employees may sit and relax; printing monthly newsletter articles on how to identify and manage various kinds of stress; establishing a "humor room" or playing comedy videotapes for employees to view during lunch and break times; and substituting for the label "stress management" a more specific label relevant to individual needs, such as one or more of the following.

Issue/need	Title
Parenting	Positive directions
Time management	Taking charge of your life
Expecting a baby	New beginnings
Helplessness	Asserting yourself
Depression	Getting a new perspective
Elder care	Giving and receiving

See appendix B for an overview of sample presentation outlines on stress management and other topics addressed in this chapter.

What Would You Do?

Suppose you have recently been hired by a midsize manufacturing company. Despite the worksite's clean exterior and neat appearance, your environmental assessment reveals that the work environment is very unhealthy because of wide-scale smoking, vending machines filled with junk food, and cramped work areas.

Your supervisor asks you to recommend changes to improve the work environment. Considering that you are the newest (and probably youngest) employee, which of the three challenges would you tackle first? Why? Describe and justify your strategy.

7

HEALTHY LIFESTYLE
PROGRAMS AND RESOURCES

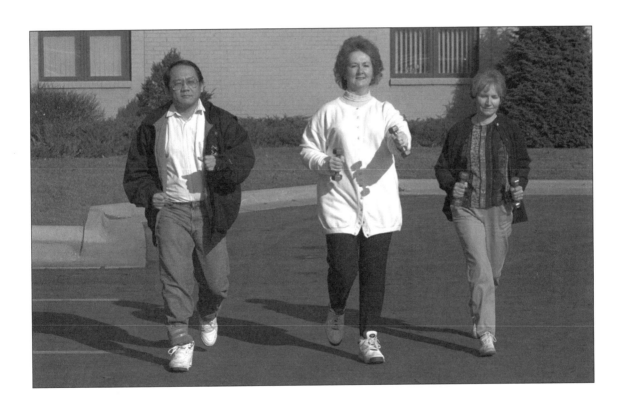

Each worksite has unique needs that require particular worksite health promotion programs and resources. The first part of this chapter presents an overview of various WHP programs, including physical fitness; back health; nutrition education and weight control; prenatal health; smoking cessation; and AIDS education and HIV prevention. The second half of the chapter covers ideas and strategies to consider when selecting resources for your WHP programs.

PHYSICAL FITNESS PROGRAMS

One of the most pressing challenges facing WHP program directors today is how to motivate employees to exercise and become physically fit. The 1996 *Surgeon General's Report on Physical Activity and Health* advises people to do at least 30 minutes a day of moderate exercise (e.g., walking at 3 to 4 miles per hour). Currently, less than 20 percent of American adults meet this standard. For the first time in the history of the United States, the percentage of inactive adults exceeds the percentage of active adults, and this startling statistic extends to the workplace.

In hopes of motivating employees to shape up, many employers now provide worksite physical fitness programs (PFPs). Some of the factors behind management's push for PFPs include the following:

- Growing evidence showing regular exercise reduces the risk of heart disease (the leading cause of death in the U.S.), stroke, and many other circulatory disorders

- Growing frustration of paying billions of dollars to treat many illnesses and disorders that are influenced largely by lifestyle

- Efforts to regain a competitive edge by improving employee health

- Growing evidence showing exercisers often outperforming their nonexercising co-workers

- An increase in the number of job applicants inquiring about fitness center or health club benefits

PROGRAM OPTIONS

While some of today's more publicized PFPs operate in modern, state-of-the-art fitness centers, most worksites do not have the need or financial resources to construct such elaborate facilities. Many of these sites instead provide small, on-site fitness centers. (See the profile on Healthworks in chapter 8 [p. 121] for an illustration of how one company makes the best use of available space for its fitness facility.) Other companies subsidize employee memberships to local health club facilities. Of course, some worksites combine strategies within their health-management framework, sometimes taking a "cafeteria plan" approach to better meet the diverse needs of their employees. (See the profile on the SAS Institute in chapter 8 [p. 120] for more details on a company that applies a multistrategy approach toward health management.)

EQUIPMENT AND FACILITY CONSIDERATIONS

Designing and equipping a healthy worksite requires considerable planning and coordination among the company and outside vendors. Considering today's options, a company needs to look closely at its budget and the marketplace; review product literature; and consult with other worksite personnel. Some of your early decisions about facility planning and purchasing equipment could make or break your program, so research as much as you need before making a choice.

PURCHASING EQUIPMENT

Equipment costs vary widely, depending on brand name, durability, computerized features, and shipping expense. In general, stationary bikes cost from $300 to $3,000; multistation weight systems go for $1,000 and up; stair climbing machines cost from $1,000 to $4,000; rowers cost $300 to $1,500; and treadmills run from $400 to $5,000. With such a huge range in quality and price of equipment, it's foolish not to shop around. Here are some tips for purchasing equipment:

- Buy equipment designed for institutional use.

- To cut costs, buy from a local firm or manufacturer whenever possible.

- To save approximately 50 percent off the retail price, buy carpet directly from the manufacturing mill.

- Ask distributors if they provide free equipment instruction.

- Buy mechanized equipment when feasible as some computerized equipment is often high maintenance.

- Check a firm's stock inventory, credit plan, warranty, and service contract. Ask if the manufacturer has product liability insurance.

- Ask salespeople for the names of other companies that have purchased the equipment and solicit opinions before buying.

- Invite sales representatives to visit your worksite to discuss your particular needs.

MAINTAINING FITNESS EQUIPMENT

The durability of a fitness facility and equipment is best preserved by maintaining a temperature near 70 degrees and humidity lower than 50 percent. Ask exercisers to put a towel over computer control panels to protect them from perspiration. Place electronic equipment in locations with adequate ventilation to reduce heat overload. Monitor equipment use to ensure that it is being used properly. As misuse is probably the biggest contributor to broken or malfunctioning equipment, you may want to hold training sessions to show how the equipment should and should not be used.

FURNISHINGS

Fans help the air-conditioning system circulate air more efficiently; large ceiling fans are more attractive than floor models. Mirrors should be shatterproof, especially in the weight room.

Mirrors give the best visual feedback when they are positioned on only two walls rather than around the room. Large standing plants, such as parlor palms, positioned in corners provide a natural look.

LIGHTING

When properly positioned, windows provide natural, inexpensive lighting. Ideally, windows should be positioned to absorb sunlight for solar heat during winter months without causing glare. Select lighting panels that provide dim lighting during off-peak hours (cuts energy consumption). Mercuryvapor, fluorescent bulbs work well for racquetball and basketball. Avoid surface-mounted fluorescent lights, as they cause glare. If you have locker rooms, recessed fluorescent lighting provides a nice ambience.

LOCKER ROOMS AND SHOWERS

Efficient ventilation in the shower room is essential for providing comfort, containing heating and cooling costs, and maintaining the overall health of the facility. A HVAC (heating, ventilating, and air conditioning) system that provides ventilation at least 40 cubic feet per minute is necessary to minimize excessive heat and moisture in showers and locker rooms.

If your company can afford lockers, full-size lockers are desirable to hang dresses and suits, whereas stacked lockers are adequate for leisure clothing. A good locker has vents for air circulation, is easy to clean, is purchased from a reputable manufacturer, includes a service contract, and can be purchased at a discount when bought in bulk.

FACILITY SURFACES

Many experts recommend surfacing your facility with a wood spring-coil floor or a polyurethane mixed foam floor with padding or carpeting treated with Scotchgard® to prevent mildew. Rubber is also popular; though it is slightly more expensive than carpet or wood, it lasts longer. The cost per square foot for synthetic foam generally runs from $4.50 to $10, good carpeting from $3.50 to $5.00, wood from $8 to $15, and rubber from $9 to $17. If your site will include a basketball court, the best surface is polyurethane-finished wood (maple, beech, or birch) pure polyurethane (such as ChemTurf), or polyurethane with acrylic resin. Prices for these surfaces run from $10 to $15 per square foot. For a racquetball court, choose a wood surface of maple, beech, or birch, costing from $10 to $15. For high-traffic surfaces, the best choice is a synthetic fiber carpeting of nylon or olefin, which runs from $5 to $10 per square foot. To avoid fraying, unraveling, and packing down, select a cut-pile version with a low pile height and tight gauge construction. Choose "action backing" over jute backing to avoid moisture buildup and mildew. In the weight room, the best surface is high-quality wood. Rubber mats (with trip-free beveled edging) should be placed under each piece of equipment and in the free-weight area to absorb sound and cushion dropped weights.

In the locker room area (if your company can afford this luxury), carpeting provides comfort, economy, safety, and easy maintenance. The carpet should have antifungus protection and be regularly wet-vacuumed and treated with Scotchgard. The color or pattern should minimize stains. In the shower and drying area of the locker room, the best shower surface is slightly abrasive, nonslip tile. Tiles set in mortar are less likely to fall out than tiles glued to water-proof gypsum board. Soft brown is a popular color and doesn't show stains as much as white. Shower walls should be tiled and epoxy-sealed. Epoxy-sealant is relatively inexpensive and can be steam-cleaned.

If you're lucky enough to afford a facility with an indoor track, choose synthetic surfaces such as rubber or a vinyl laminated to a sponge-rubber cushion. Latex, full-poured urethane, and vented urethane also work well. Corners should be banked slightly to minimize stress on the lower leg. (Remind runners to alternate direction on a daily basis to reduce musculoskeletal stress on one side of the body.)

If your company plans an outdoor fitness trail, your best selections for surface materials are decomposed granite, limestone quarry screenings, crushed coral, or woodchips. In constructing a trail, cut a 3.5-inch deep trough with a landscaping tractor. The dirt wells up on the sides of the trough, creating a natural border that holds the surface material in place. Fill the trough with 2 inches of compacted gravel and top it with a surface material, making the trail level with the ground. Locate the trail away from office buildings so workers are not distracted by passersby. For one-way traffic only, a 4-foot path is adequate. You'll need a 7-foot path or bigger for two-way traffic. Provide distance markers and perhaps a bench or par course along the trail.

Back Health

Back injury is one of the most common on-the-job injuries at the worksite. In fact, nearly 25 percent of all workers' compensation claims are classified as musculoskeletal injuries, with low back injury being the most common. Nearly 2 percent of the U.S. work force files a low back injury claim each year. A minor low back (muscular) strain costs an employer about $400 per injury. More serious back injuries such as a bulging disk or fractured vertebrae often cost $5,000 each.

By establishing on-site programs, many companies are reducing the incidence and cost of low back injuries. Research indicates that the most successful low back programs include three major components:

- Prevention and health promotion
- Intervention and treatment for injured employees
- Rehabilitation and a return-to-work protocol

Treating and rehabilitating injured workers is usually provided by occupational health nurses, physical therapists, massage therapists, and other allied health care personnel, but the WHP professional often plays a major role in the promotion of back health.

Occupational Injuries

Some researchers who contend that most occupational injuries are caused by a combination of environmental (worksite) and personal factors question whether it is really appropriate to expect a single intervention to reduce the risk of such injuries. Apparently, some companies agree with this notion and provide multiple interventions in an attempt to prevent worksite injuries. For example, Fitzler and Berger studied the impact of a multifaceted low back program on the incidence of low back injuries and costs. The program consisted of three components:

1. **Prevention**—low back education and awareness activities
2. **Intervention**—reporting low back pain and injury immediately
3. **Treatment**—protocols ranging from heat applications to mild analgesics

Considering the program's emphasis on encouraging employees to report low back injuries immediately, the authors were not surprised to see the number of low back injuries increase from 20 to 34 in the first 24 months of the program. Yet the number of low back injuries that resulted in lost work time dropped from 10 to 6 injuries, and the frequency rate dropped nearly 50 percent—from 2.78 injuries per 100 employees to 1.56 in less than 2 years. Moreover, workers' compensation costs for low back injuries dropped tenfold, from $200,000 to about $14,000 in the same time frame.

PREVENTION OF BACK INJURIES

Perhaps the most effective incentive to promote healthy backs at the worksite is constant support from management, supervisors, and co-workers. Here are some ideas for promoting healthy practices at your worksite:

• **Awareness and knowledge.** Make employees aware of the risk of low back injuries by providing company and industry-specific data; teaching the structure and function of the spine and lower back; and providing instructions on how to identify high-risk tasks by showing slides and/or videotapes of employees performing work functions. Important learning and behavioral concepts can be reinforced with poster campaigns, paycheck stuffers, monthly safety meetings, and other high visibility methods. Display posters of easy stretching routines at key locations. Use the company newsletter to illustrate spinal anatomy and tips on proper body mechanics for lifting, pulling, and pushing.

• **Practice.** A trained leader teaches employees proper body mechanics for lifting, bending, carrying, pushing, pulling, and reaching; employees practice prework stretching and strengthening routines daily with their immediate supervisor.

• **Implementation/follow-up.** All employees are trained to lead their co-workers in daily prework stretching and strengthening exercises. Consider using extrinsic incentives to encourage employee participation in prework stretching and warm-up routines. For example, injury-free employees at designated intervals (3, 6, 9, and 12 months) can enter a sweepstakes to win one or more prizes presented at the company holiday party at the end of the year.

NUTRITION EDUCATION AND WEIGHT CONTROL

Consider that . . . over half of all American workers are overweight; about two-thirds of American workers eat unhealthy diets; a high-fat diet is a major risk factor for health problems associated with many health care claims (circulatory, digestive, cancer, and metabolic); and overweight people have significantly longer hospital stays and file more health care

---

WORKSITE PROGRAMS AND THEIR IMPACT—BACK INJURY PREVENTION

What impact can an on-site back injury prevention program have on employees? Here are a few examples of the payoff in some organizations:

• **Biltrite Corporation (Chelsea, MA)**—Within 1 year of operation, the company's back program produced a 90 percent drop ($150,000 savings) in back injury claims requiring compensation.

• **Capital Wire and Cable (Plano, TX)**—The company saved more than $83,000 within 20 months of instituting a new low back program.

• **Coca-Cola (Atlanta, GA)**—Bottle plant employees perform a 10-minute pre-work routine to prepare for the rigors of loading and unloading trucks. Accidents have decreased 83 percent and produced a yearly savings of over $250 per employee in lost time and replacement costs.

• **Lockheed Missile and Space Company (Sunnyvale, CA)**—The company reported a 67.5 percent drop in low back injury costs within 14 months of implementing its low back program.

• **Pepsi-Cola Bottling Plants (Riviera Beach and Pompano Beach, FL)**—The company reported that low back injuries dropped from 146 to 13 within 2 years of a mandatory pre-work stretching program.

claims than their co-workers. Given all this, it's little wonder that nutrition and weight control are prime target areas for WHP.

ENVIRONMENTAL STRATEGIES

WHP personnel can promote healthier eating for employees in several ways:

- Distribute nutrition education materials in the cafeteria and near canteens, vending machines, or break areas.

- Offer heart-healthy entrees, a salad bar, and other healthy options.

- Affix "healthy choice" labels to foods low in fat, calories, sugar, salt, and cholesterol.

- Offer a weekly menu of nutritious bag lunches that employees can prepare.

- Offer discounted prices on "healthy heart" entrees.

- Ease out the junk food from vending machines and replace with fruits, fruit juices, low-fat dairy products, and other nutritious foods. (Do not try to get rid of all junk food at once!)

- Place weight scales in company restrooms for employees to regularly monitor their weight.

- Provide free body fat measurements several times each month; skinfold calipers are relatively inexpensive.

PROGRAMMING

Consider your options and goals before committing to purchase program resources. For example, a multifaceted program of screenings, exercise sessions, competitions, and follow-up counseling sessions may be a cost-effective approach to impact high-risk employees with multiple health problems. Weight-control programs may consist of small group sessions, large group lectures, self-management tips, or weight-loss competitions.

Timing is an important consideration to promote healthy eating. For example, lunchtime is a good opportunity to offer lunch 'n learn seminars on such issues as cholesterol reduction, hypertension control, and diabetes control. March is national nutrition month in the U.S., an excellent time to introduce new programs for workers shaping up for the summer.

PRENATAL HEALTH PROMOTION

Nationwide, employers pay approximately $3,500 per full-term pregnancy and delivery without complications. A pregnancy with complications can cost an employer *several hundred thousand dollars*; of course, some of this expense is eventually passed

WORKSITE PROGRAMS AND THEIR IMPACT—WEIGHT LOSS

What impact can a weight-reduction/nutrition program have on employees? Here are some examples:

- **Lycoming County, PA**—Three independent weight-loss competitions between various industries and banks in Lycoming County, Pennsylvania, produced an average weight loss of 12 pounds per participant.

- **Campbell's Soup Company**—Two hundred thirty-three employee participants in Campbell's STRIP (Spare Tire Reduction Incentive Program) lost 3,078 pounds within 3 months.

- **Du Pont**—Du Pont's weight loss program produced an average weight loss of 5.5 pounds per participant, with 85 percent of those maintaining their losses at least 3 months.

- **L.L. Bean Company**—Seventy percent of the 77 Heart Club members at L.L. Bean had 14 percent lower cholesterol levels within 8 months, which cut their heart disease risk by 28 percent.

- **Lockheed Missile and Space Company**—Employees lost a total of 14,378 pounds in the company's 3-month "Take It Off" program, at a cost of only 94 cents per lost pound.

- **Scherer Brothers Lumber**—This company of 150 employees made its environment healthier by removing candy machines and adding fruit dispensers, replacing caffeinated coffee with decaf, and offering healthy snacks free of charge.

FINANCIAL IMPACT OF PREGNANCY COMPLICATIONS

To understand the financial impact of pregnancy-related complications on some employers, consider what happened at two Oster-Sunbeam worksites. In 1 year, four severely ill babies were born to employees at one worksite; medical care costs for the four infants totaled $500,000. The next year at the other plant, three more babies were born prematurely; one infant's lengthy hospitalization exhausted the company's major medical coverage. Soon after, the company established a prenatal program that has slashed the average cost per birth by 90 percent. Within a year of establishing the new prenatal health education program, costs per maternity case at the Coushatta, Louisiana, plant dropped from $27,242 to $2,893; the cost per case at the Holly Springs, Mississippi, plant dropped from $3,500 to $2,872. Moreover, only one premature birth has occurred at either plant since the start of the program.

on to employees through higher insurance premiums, deductibles, and copayments.

Statistics show the percentage of unhealthy infants born in the United States is a nationwide problem. The U.S. infant death rate is higher than it is in 17 other industrialized nations. (One in 100 American newborns will die during his or her first year of life.) One of every 14 American babies is born with a low birth weight, and the medical bills for these infants costs over $3 billion a year. The hospital bill for one premature infant can be $500,000, whereas a baby born with breathing or feeding problems may require more than $60,000 of health care services a month! Given these numbers, and that much of the expense is passed on to businesses in the form of increased insurance premiums, it only makes sense that WHP develop aggressive programs on prenatal care.

GENERAL RECOMMENDATIONS

One of the most ambitious worksite-based prenatal health promotion initiatives, the Southern Regional Corporate Coalition to Improve Maternal and Child Health, consists of 29 employers from 17 southern states. Coalition studies suggest that companies will have a healthier and more productive workforce as well as cut their own expenses if they do the following:

1. Include a maternal and infant health benefit in their insurance packages, with incentives to encourage families to use preventive services such as prenatal care for pregnant women.

2. Review their maternity leave policies and grant leave for pregnant women, without compromising a successful return to work.

3. Engage in public-private partnerships to develop health care public policy and encourage good maternal health.

4. Provide educational programs for employees and their families on preventive health care for mothers and children.

Items 1 through 3 here generally are the concern of human resources and benefits managers. But WHP personnel are often responsible for writing and implementing educational programs on prenatal, infant, maternal, and child health.

A PRENATAL HEALTH EDUCATION PROGRAM

A typical prenatal health education program consists of the following components:

• **Pre-pregnancy counseling**. Employees interested in learning about their genetic predisposition are encouraged to meet with an occupational health nurse to discuss influential factors, for example, age, family history, lifestyle, and health status on pregnancy.

• **Identification**. Employees who believe they are pregnant are asked to visit the company's on-site nurse for a pregnancy (urine) test.

• **Referral**. If an employee is pregnant, she is informed of the company's health care benefits and encouraged to visit her personal physician; to qualify for maternity health care benefits, pregnant employees/dependents are required to attend on-site prenatal health education classes.

• **Education classes**. In conjunction with regular visits to their personal physicians (or on-site physician), pregnant women participate in the company's prenatal health education program taught by a certified professional. One-hour programs are offered every 2 weeks on company time, and typically include two phases.

1. **Information phase:** prenatal care, nutrition, substance use and abuse, discomforts of pregnancy, fetal development, signs and symptoms of labor and birthing, and recommendations of postnatal home care.

2. **Clinical phase:** one-on-one screenings and discussions to assess each woman's blood pressure, weight, water retention level, and urine test results.

In between classes, informal sessions are held for women who are in the later stages of pregnancy or are considered high risk because of excess weight, hypertension, or a history of difficult childbirth.

The Colorado Department of Health Affairs estimates that a minimum of $9 could be saved for every dollar spent on prenatal care. If long-term costs were included, the savings could be as much as $11 for every dollar spent. Numerous companies including Cigna, First Chicago Bank, and Sunbeam/Oster have reported impressive cost savings from their prenatal health education programs.

MOTIVATING PARTICIPATION

A high participation level of pregnant employees (especially those at risk) is vital to the overall success of any prenatal health education program. Although many companies have mandatory participation policies (to qualify for maternity benefits), employees tend to take a more genuine interest in prenatal programs that include personal incentives. Some of the more successful incentives include:

- offering programs on company time

- waiving the first year health insurance deductible if the expectant mother attends all scheduled prenatal classes

- offering monetary rewards—$100, for example—for attending all prenatal classes and screening sessions

- paying a higher percentage (90 percent vs. 50 percent, for example) of the health care bill for participating mothers

Since the actual effectiveness of incentives will vary from worksite to worksite, incentives should be tailored around employees needs and interests,

the worksite culture, and an employer's financial situation.

Companies are discovering that investing in prenatal and maternal health programs pays off. Each high-risk pregnancy that is avoided saves tens, if not hundreds, of thousands of dollars for employers and society, and translates into a healthier work force in the future.

SMOKING CONTROL POLICIES AND PROGRAMS

One of the most visible examples of business' commitment to employees' health is reflected in the growth of smoking control policies at many worksites. Nearly two-thirds of all medium and large worksites have official smoking control policies and smoking cessation programs with more expected to follow into the new millennium.

WHY TARGET SMOKING?

Many factors are responsible for business' growing push for smoke-free worksites. First, federal agencies are addressing the issue in several ways. The U.S. Surgeon General's Report attributes an estimated 420,000 deaths each year to cigarette smoking, making it America's number one cause of preventable death; in 1986, the General Services Administration (GSA) significantly restricted smoking in 6,800 federal office buildings; and in 1990, the Environmental Protection Agency (EPA) officially classified second-hand smoke as a significant indoor pollutant and a class-A carcinogen. Second, many antidrug campaigns are spreading into worksites and targeting illegal drugs as well as legal drugs such as cigarettes (nicotine). Third, more nonsmokers are requesting their employers to establish smoke-free working environments. Fourth, more business owners are becoming aware of the economic costs of smoking employees; smokers are absent 2 to 5 days more per year than nonsmokers and incur approximately 15 percent higher health care costs than nonsmokers. Fifth, there is a growing body of statutory, regulatory, and judicial developments that

- grant employees the right to sue employers if smoking is permitted in a workplace,

- stipulate that employers can be held partially accountable for employee pain, discomfort, and illness caused by smoke in the workplace, and

- rule that there are no legal grounds for claims that smoking at work is a constitutional right.

Additional factors influencing worksite smoking control efforts include ensuring the purity of manufactured products, preventing property and equipment damage, and enhancing a company's corporate image to shareholders and the public (see table 7.1).

PROGRAM AND POLICY PLANNING

When planning a smoking control policy, a program director should properly structure and communicate its strategy for establishing smoke-free initiatives at the worksite. For example, more worksites are integrating their smoke-free efforts within "clean air" policy proposals and the theme of protecting the health of employees. This minimizes the potential for heated debates, personal conflicts, and friction between smoking employees and management.

So-called "half-and-half" policies (i.e., banning smoking only at work stations) are counterproductive, as they force smokers to leave their work areas to smoke, resulting in lost productivity. In contrast, a total "clean air" worksite policy can eliminate such violations and also help smokers trying to quit. Removing all cigarette vending machines from the worksite and providing stop-smoking programs with financial rewards also helps smokers quit.

An excellent time to implement stop-smoking activities and policy changes is during the Great American Smokeout sponsored by the American Cancer Society each November. Reportedly, some employers give employees 6 months' notice before implementing a no-smoking policy.

Table 7.1 The Economic Costs of Cigarette Smoking to Employers in 1976 and 2000		
Cost category	**1976**	**2000 (projected)**
Lost production	$19,139,800,000	$49,061,129,055
Direct health care	8,224,000,000	46,653,716,256
Total	**$27,363,800,000**	**$95,714,854,311**

1976 costs provided by the *New England Journal of Medicine* (vol. 11, no. 298, 1978). Year 2000 cost estimates provided by Health Management Associates; lost production costs based on 4 percent annual inflation; direct health care costs based on 7.5 percent annual medical care inflation.

SMOKING CONTROL POLICY BENEFITS

Potential benefits to employers who establish smoking control policies include, but are not limited to:

- lower health-life-fire insurance and workers' compensation premium costs
- fewer health care claims and costs due to smoking-related conditions
- less absenteeism due to smoking-related illnesses
- less property and equipment damage and maintenance costs due to cigarette smoking
- fewer accidents and reduced fire risk
- greater productivity (avoidance of "downtime" used for smoking breaks)
- fewer premature disabilities and deaths due to cigarette smoking

Actual benefits depend largely on factors such as the extent of smoking control measures; the amount of smoking and biological damage to the heart, lungs, and blood vessels before such measures are implemented; the percentage of employees who smoke off site; the general health of workers; and co-exposure to other occupational hazards such as asbestos, coal dust, etc.

On-site smoking cessation programs have been found to exist most commonly in large companies (more than 1,000 employees), but have better success rates in smaller worksites (fewer than 250 employees). Facilitators are easily identified and social relationships within the worksite tend to be stronger than in larger, dispersed worksites. In larger worksites, employees from the same department should be placed in the same smoking-cessation groups to maintain interpersonal relationships and group cohesiveness. Starting a support group of ex-smokers is often helpful to encourage recent quitters to keep it up.

By examining the demographics of your organization, and reviewing health risk appraisal data, you will be able to compare your workforce's smoking rate and note whether the subgroups mentioned earlier match your experience; consequently, you can then decide whether to apply the percentage rate by the respective subgroups.

The three general elements of a successful intervention program are:

1. consistent and repeated advice from a team of providers to quit smoking,

2. setting a specific quit date, and

3. providing follow-up visits.

Additional modalities specifically for physicians include:

- Support and mention of current programs offered at the worksite or in conjunction with the health care provider organization.

- Referral to community group counseling.

- Advice from more than one clinician (if available).

- Using chart reminders to identify those who smoke.

Interventions provided at the worksite or by the health care provider organization should contain the option of three core elements. A combination of these three elements may not be the best for all smokers; however, to increase the probability of gaining a higher success and reduced relapse rate, the combination of these three strategies should be considered.

The first strategy centers around education and counseling. The education component should focus on the health effects of smoking, the importance of gaining support at work and at home, and moving the individual to the action phase (i.e., setting a quit date). Once an individual is in the action phase, the counselor should work through the following priorities:

- build readiness to quit

- build support needed to quit

- build skills needed to quit

- identify a quit date

- assess success at various time intervals depending on the client after quit date

- prevent relapse

The second strategy centers around a nicotine replacement product. A nicotine replacement product should be used in combination with the counseling once the quit date is reached. When used correctly and in combination with education and counseling, nicotine replacement products increase long-term smoking cessation rates by about one-third. A 4-milligram (mg) dose of the nicotine replacement product seems to be more effective than the 2-mg dose in highly nicotine-dependent clients. The evidence suggests that nicotine replacement products are most effective in combination with continuous counseling. Clients should receive proper instruction on how to use these products as part of the on-going counseling.

At this time, there seems to be limited evidence that a third type of intervention strategy should be used in combination with the education/counseling and nicotine replacement strategies.

The third strategy centers around Zyban sustained-released tablets, a non-nicotine aid for smoking cessation. Initially developed and marketed as an antidepressant, Zyban affects the part of the brain that inhibits addictive behavior. The effectiveness of Zyban as an aid for smoking cessation was demonstrated in two placebo-controlled, double-blind trials in nondepressed cigarette smokers. In these studies, Zyban was used in conjunction with individual smoking cessation counseling. Initial results indicate that Zyban is a successful smoking cessation intervention in nearly 50 percent of all users.

Self-help interventions (written materials in particular) generally produce low initial quit rates, but are effective in helping quitters sustain their efforts and assisting nonquitters to make additional attempts. The American Lung Association's self-help guide, Freedom From Smoking, and the follow-up version, A Lifetime of Freedom From Smoking, are designed for employees wanting to quit on their own.

Group cessation methods (multicomponent behaviorally based programs) often produce 1-year quit rates of 30 percent to 40 percent, but often attract a small percentage of employees.

In contrast, incentive and competition-based programs may attract good participation and produce favorable quit rates; however, these programs are typically based on self-reported behavior that should be verified with biochemical measures such as thiocyanate or carbon monoxide testing. In a survey of over 200 adult smokers, respondents preferred smoking cessation programs that included

- ways to remain smoke free for life,
- an endorsement by doctors,
- ways to deal with potential weight gain,
- a list of relaxation techniques to use while quitting, and
- a list of healthy substitutes for smoking.

When evaluating the impact of worksite smoking-cessation programs, it's important to define quit rate, long-term abstinence, and any other key terms or concepts that can be subjectively quantified. **Quit rate** is commonly defined as a percent or ratio of the number of successful employees quitting to the number of employees who started the intervention. A minimum period of a year is generally accepted for judging long-term abstinence. Also, be wary of vendors and proposals promising quit rates of more than 50 percent. Ask vendors for the names and phone numbers of past and current clients who can verify such claims.

A Sample Schedule for Implementing a Smoke-free Policy

Below we'll describe a step-by-step plan for organizations wanting to expand a partial restriction policy into a total smoke-free environmental policy.

Months 1–3

In the first month, form a smoking issues committee consisting of managers and labor representatives who are nonsmokers, smokers, and ex-smokers. Consider hiring an outside consultant to facilitate committee meetings and phases of the project.

In months 2 and 3, study the smoking issue by reviewing the company's current policies, other companies' policies, local and state ordinances, federal laws (EPA and OSHA, for example), and legal liability with a corporate attorney.

Months 4–5

In the fourth month, survey employee attitudes and behaviors relevant to smoking. Develop a simple

Worksite Programs and Their Impact—Smoking Control

These examples from well-known companies illustrate potential benefits of smoking control programs and policies.

- **Speedcall Corporation (Hayward, CA)**—After the company's president offered each employee a $7 weekly bonus for not smoking at the worksite, the number of smoking employees dropped from 24 to 5 within a year.
- **Dow Chemical (Texas Division)**—Twenty-four percent of the company's smokers competed in a smoking-cessation competition. Those quitting for at least 1 year entered a raffle for a fishing boat. At prize time, nearly 80 percent of the entrants were smoke free.
- **UNUM Life Insurance Company (Portland, ME)**—The company reported an estimated health care cost savings of $200,000 in the first year of its worksite smoking ban.
- **Pacific Bell (Seattle, WA)**—The percentage of smoking employees dropped from 28 percent to 20 percent within 2 years of its worksite smoking ban. Visits to the company's health clinic for respiratory problems dropped 13 percent, and respiratory-based absences dropped 20 percent.

questionnaire to assess employee attitudes toward a smoking policy. An easy six-point scale could be used:

1. No smoking restrictions at all

2. Designate several smoking areas

3. Designate one smoking area

4. Ban smoking indoors

5. Start a completely smoke-free workplace

6. Do not hire smokers (a policy prohibited in some states)

During the fifth month, develop a draft of the proposed policy. Review employee responses and construct a policy for a preliminary review by senior management. If the policy is not accepted, revise it accordingly and resubmit it.

MONTHS 6–9

Use the sixth month to obtain mainstream support. Meet with key supervisors and middle managers to inform them of the policy and to encourage their support.

Announce the new policy in the seventh month by sending a memo from the human resources or personnel department to inform all employees of the purpose of the policy and the dates it will gradually go into effect.

During the eighth month, implement partial restrictions to reflect the locations cited in the survey. For example, restrict smoking to designated break areas only. This is also a good time to remove all cigarette machines from the worksite.

Devote the ninth month to educating employees on the hazards and costs of smoking. Use several communication methods (e.g., newsletter, message boards, health fair) to inform employees of the health risks and financial costs of smoking.

MONTHS 10–12

Over the next 3 months, begin to offer smoking-cessation programs to interested employees and spouses. Review the section on Program and Policy Planning earlier in the chapter to determine appropriate interventions, participation fee policy, program schedules, and incentives.

Now is the time to send a memo to all employees outlining the entire policy and reminding them of the dates the policy will go into effect. The policy can now be implemented with clearly defined protocols on monitoring.

Schedule monthly meetings over the next 6 months to solicit committee members' feedback on the new policy. See appendix A for smoking control resources.

AIDS EDUCATION AND HIV DISEASE PREVENTION

Acquired Immunodeficiency Syndrome (AIDS) remains a large health problem. As of 1998, the Centers for Disease Control estimates that nearly a million Americans are infected with HIV (Human Immunodeficiency Virus). Other sobering statistics reflect the seriousness of this disease:

• Although men are stricken in greater numbers, women are contracting HIV at a proportionately higher rate.

• More than 14 million American women—many heterosexual—will contract HIV early in the third millennium.

Since 1 of every 250 Americans has HIV, many American worksites have at least one employee who is HIV positive. Workers in health care settings dealing with body fluids are particularly at risk. Thus, such facilities have developed regulations in response to Healthy People 2000 Objective 18.14, which stipulates that regulations to protect workers from exposure to blood-borne infections, including HIV infection, should extend to all facilities where workers are at risk of occupational transmission of HIV.

Despite the significant growth in worksite efforts to educate employees on HIV and AIDS, numerous questions remain to be adequately addressed at many worksites.

THE ECONOMIC COST OF HIV/AIDS

Until the early 1990s, the average life expectancy of a person with HIV/AIDS was projected to be about 2 years; the estimated cost of "lifetime" hospital care for an infected individual can be as high as $60,000, and as high as $100,000 for total health care costs, according to the CDC. However, medical treatment for persons with HIV disease is steadily improving, enhancing the quality of life for those diagnosed with the disease. In fact, HIV disease in the United States is gradually changing from being considered a terminal illness to being viewed as a chronic, treatable illness, at least in some cases. Thus, the increasing number of people with HIV disease will live longer and, in many cases, continue to work. Consequently, more employers are paying the increasing costs for their medical insurance and disability pay.

Some employers are already feeling the crunch of HIV-AIDS through higher insurance costs associated with HIV-related claims. In fact, productivity losses due to HIV-related illnesses and premature deaths are more than $125 billion per year. Nonetheless, HIV-related health care costs still contribute far less to the nation's rising health care cost index than other factors such as cost-shifting, high technology, medical inflation, higher utilization, and medical malpractice insurance premiums.

Faced with the rising health care costs of HIV-AIDS treatment, more companies and insurers are betting on managed care programs to help slow these cost increases. Of course, the key to managed care for HIV disease is to reduce inpatient hospitalization, which is the most expensive component of traditional AIDS care. Case management (individualized care at home or in an outpatient facility) is the most common type of managed care used in treating HIV disease; it is capable of saving as much as $50,000 per case, according to some insurers. Furthermore, home care treatment is less expensive, more psychologically comforting, and less likely to expose the patient to other diseases that are in a hospital setting. This type of managed care approach certainly merits consideration as a cost-control strategy. Yet, to effectively deal with this complex and evolving phenomenon, companies will have to establish employee education and prevention activities that appeal to as many employees as possible, especially to those in greatest need.

WHAT CAN A COMPANY DO?

To date, numerous companies, including Syntex, Bank of America, AT&T, Eaton, Transamerica, and Pacific Telesis, have developed personnel policies to deal with HIV disease in the workplace. Bank of America is one of the most progressive companies in this area; it makes certain accommodations (flexible work hours, for example) for an employee with HIV disease, as long as the person's condition does not impair the department's efficiency. Another progressive step is treating HIV-AIDS just like any other serious disease and allowing an infected employee to work as long as his or her health permits.

WORKSITE AIDS EDUCATION

It is estimated that 50,000 people in the U.S. die yearly from AIDS complications. According to Dr. C. Everett Koop, former U.S. Surgeon General, with proper information and education, as many as 14,000 people could be saved yearly. A growing number of companies are responding to this challenge.

Ideally, employers should address the issue of HIV infection before the first case is reported at the worksite, when the employees' level of objectivity and receptivity is probably the greatest. Waiting to educate employees on HIV-AIDS issues after a co-worker has been infected may only intensify general hysteria throughout a work force.

Employers who have made a corporate commitment to provide HIV education have received favorable response from employees, especially when information and education has been integrated into existing health benefits and internal communications.

The Business Leadership Task Force, comprised of 15 major northern California employers, has taken a leadership role in providing HIV education at worksites since 1983. A number of task force members such as AT&T, Bank of America, Chevron, Levi Strauss, Mervyn's Department Stores, Pacific Telesis, and Wells Fargo have developed a videotape, "An Epidemic of Fear," for use in corporate HIV information and education campaigns. In addition, several task force member companies provide the following:

- lectures for managers by HIV experts
- HIV information classes for employees, workers with HIV, and their relatives
- HIV-related articles in company newsletters
- video presentations that employees may borrow for home viewing

RESPONDING TO AIDS: TEN PRINCIPLES FOR THE WORKPLACE

The Citizens' Commission on AIDS for New York City and Northern New Jersey has drafted guidelines to help employers manage AIDS in the workplace. *Responding to AIDS: Ten Principles for the Workplace* has been endorsed by more than 370 companies and organizations. The principles are as follows:

1. People with AIDS or HIV infection at any stage are entitled to the same rights and opportunities as people with other serious or life-threatening illnesses.

2. Employment policies must comply with federal, state, and local laws and regulations.

3. Employment policies should be based on the scientific and epidemiological evidence that people who are HIV-positive or who have AIDS cannot transmit the virus to co-workers through ordinary workplace contact.

4. The highest levels of management and union leadership should unequivocally endorse nondiscriminatory employment policies and educational programs about HIV disease.

5. Employers and unions should communicate their support of these policies to workers in simple, clear, and unambiguous terms.

6. Employers should provide employees with sensitive, accurate, and up-to-date information about risk reduction in their personal lives.

7. Employers have a duty to protect the confidentiality of employees' medical information.

8. To prevent work disruption and rejection by co-workers of an employee with AIDS or HIV infection, employers and unions should educate all employees before such an incident occurs and as needed thereafter.

9. Employers should not require HIV screening as part of pre-employment or general workplace physical examinations but can provide the phone number and location of local health department anonymous test sites.

10. In those special occupational settings where there may be a potential risk of exposure to HIV—for example, health care workers who may be exposed to blood or blood products—employers should provide ongoing education and training in universal blood and body fluid precautions as well as the necessary equipment to reinforce appropriate infection control procedures.

Although several approaches are being used at worksites, some experts feel that peer-to-peer education among employees is the most effective approach. See appendix A for a listing of AIDS/HIV education resources.

MEDICAL SELF-CARE AND HEALTH CARE CONSUMERISM

Growing concerns over higher health care costs and uncontrolled utilization in the past decade has prompted many worksites to develop medical self-care and consumerism programs. This emphasis seems well justified, since:

- The average person in the United States sees a doctor about five times a year and takes about seven different prescriptions per year.

- Over 70 percent of all visits to doctors for new health problems are probably unnecessary.

- About 11 percent of these visits are for uncomplicated (minor) colds.

- Over 80 percent of all health problems are treated at home, and an even greater number could be treated successfully with self-care.

For maximum impact, medical self-care and consumerism efforts should be directed toward both employees and their dependents; dependents' health care utilization is typically 20 percent or higher than employee utilization.

One strategy employers use is to distribute resources such as self-care books, newsletters, and videocassettes at the worksite or mail to employees' homes. These resources are designed to help individuals do the following:

- Identify when a health problem is a true emergency (since approximately 55 percent of all visits to emergency departments are not urgent).

- Learn how to use self-care measures to treat minor ailments.

- Compare health care providers on important quality and cost criteria.

- Ask the right questions of their health care providers.

- Understand cost-sharing and key features of health insurance (e.g., who pays for what [premium, deductible, and copayment], what types of alternative health care providers are in the plan).

Preliminary reports at worksites using medical self-care and consumer education interventions indicate they are saving $3 to $5 for each dollar spent on an intervention.

Medical self-care interventions operating at many multisite organizations include core communications, such as self-care books, newsletters (from you and/or the local health plan), group orientations, and other promotional materials. To support and target high-risk individuals, a telephone counseling service is one of the fastest growing options. The service is patient-advocate focused, and the goal is to assist individuals in making better health care decisions at home and with their physician. The telephone service can be part of the targeted high-risk employee process or set up independently with health plan providers. An additional service that will impact program outcomes is to use this system for chronic disease management and disability management. Essentially, the more preventive care and health services that are integrated within the organization, the more outreaching the impact. When developing and implementing such services to dispersed sites, consider the following topics for awareness campaigns or educational seminars:

- Managing high blood pressure

- Taking care of your back

- Home remedies for flu/colds

- Allergy education

- Managing diabetes

- Nutrition and exercise for diabetes

- Asthma management

- Women's and men's health issues

- How to get a preventive exam

Provide visible support and enroll the family in this activity for greatest impact. Partnering with the

QUAKER OATS HEALTH MANAGEMENT PLAN

One of the earliest worksite-based health management plans focusing on medical self-care and consumerism was implemented by The Quaker Oats Company in the early 1980s. Its integrated plan includes the following features:

- A company-produced booklet (*Informed Choices*) that helps employees and dependents decide on when to seek health care, how to compare providers on quality and cost criteria, how to select a health care provider, and what questions to ask a provider.

- Financial incentives within a health expense account in which Quaker Oats allocates a fixed amount of money (about $400) that employees can use toward their health insurance premium, deductible, and/or copayment. Unused money is applied to the following year's allocation.

- A WHP program (Live Well—Be Well) that offers health screenings, seminars, and personal health-enhancement activities.

Prior to adopting its integrated approach, Quaker's health care costs rose nearly 20 percent per year; since then, Quaker's health care costs have risen an average of about 7 percent per year.

local health plans at multisite organizations will provide you with local staff support and reduce funding of the program.

Some of the more popular self-care and consumerism resources used by employers are listed in appendix A.

PROGRAMMING RESOURCES

A major factor influencing the scope and specificity of an organization's WHP programs is resources. On-site facilities, personnel, and communication resources are only a few of the valuable entities needed to plan and operate a successful program.

LOCATION RESOURCES

In many worksites, health promotion programs and activities do not have to be confined to a single location. However, an organization's primary goals and resources largely influence the types of programs that can be feasibly implemented. Issues such as cost and effectiveness are influenced to some extent by site selection. In general, if an organization is more interested in keeping costs to an absolute minimum than achieving a high level of effectiveness, it should assess the prospect of having programs and activities conducted at off-site facilities. However, if effectiveness is most important to the organization, then it will probably benefit most from on-site programs, especially if the company has more than 500 employees. By and large, the location should be conducive to the structure, function, and goals of each program. For example, how much formal instruction will occur? Will participants be sitting or active? Will audiovisual materials be used? How much space is needed? Is privacy an issue?

FINDING ON-SITE LOCATIONS

Seminar-type programs such as stress management, nutrition, weight management, and smoking cessation are best provided in quiet, classroom-type settings with no distractions. Conference rooms, employee lounges, and cafeterias at low-usage times are also popular locations to offer such programs. For example, Sentry Corporation in Stevens Point,

Wisconsin, converted an unused area into a "quiet room" specially equipped with sofas, soft lights, and soothing music for employees to ease their stress.

As more companies decentralize, many employees find themselves working in several work settings located away from a company's main facilities. Union Pacific Railroad has given a new meaning to the term "fitness track" with its innovative approach to reaching its traveling workforce (see chapter 8, p. 114, for a profile on UP).

Efficient space utilization is particularly important for worksites with limited facilities. First, the worksite should be assessed to determine possible areas for better utilization. A feasibility grid, shown in table 7.2, can help planners determine the most efficient use of existing resources. The key is not just to use space that is already used more efficiently, but also to take advantage of unused space and quiet times.

Some smaller companies pool their finances to rent or lease a community gymnasium, swimming pool, and other facilities for employee health programs. In addition, local health clubs, fitness centers in shopping malls, and community fitness centers also should be considered by employers looking for off-site facilities. In fact, many employers pay all or some portion of membership fees so employees may use local health clubs.

PERSONNEL RESOURCES

The essence of every successful WHP program lies in the quality of its personnel. You will encounter wide variation in how much responsibility and how large a budget you are given, depending on the size of your company and your position within it. Given the programs the task force has determined are practical through the identification and assessment phases, what personnel are needed to implement the program on a practical scale, based on the overall resources of the company? If the company is large, the task force can examine the issue of whether more professional staff is needed and/or affordable. For example, depending on the budget, one of your options is to send a staff member to obtain and/or retain specific certification and other programs that are listed in chapter 10.

Regarding smaller companies that must rely on a smaller number of professional staff (sometimes only

Table 7.2 Sample Feasibility Grid Framework

	Areas				
Activity	**Medical department**	**Cafeteria**	**Fitness center**	**Conference room**	**Outside**
• Health screening	X				
• Health risk					
appraisal		X			
• Programs					
back				X	
EAP	X				
nutrition		X			
self-care		X			
lifestyle		X			
walking					X
• Physical therapy			X		
• Work hardening				X	

one) and mostly volunteers or outsourced personnel, can existing personnel be tapped? Are there people in the company with health-related expertise? For example, perhaps there is a certified aerobics instructor among the workforce. If not, would the company pay to get someone certified? Or are there other forms of certification that do not require an enormous investment but that would be useful?

Whether an organization chooses to use a professional staff, rely on in-house volunteers, or use a combination approach, it is important for staff members to work together as a team in order to reach as many employees as possible. Due to its large workforce, diverse populations, and multisite installations, Langley Air Force Base relies heavily on its WHP staff to work as a team toward achieving its primary goals. See chapter 8, page 121, for a profile on Langley's Air Force Base.

SELECTING CONSULTANTS

As many American worksites experience downsizing, aging workers, and greater efficiency demands, many employers call upon health promotion consultants to assist them in one or more of the following capacities:

Pre-Program	**Programming**	**Evaluation**
Feasibility study	Database development	Benefit-cost analysis
Conceptualization	Program planning	Cost-effectiveness analysis
Staff development	Incentives design	Break-even analysis
Break-even analysis	Marketing	
Facility design	Integration	
Equipment purchase and layout	Promotion and benefits	
Health claims data analysis		

Since few organizations really know about a consultant's capabilities until a project is actually underway, selecting a consultant should be approached with a great deal of consideration to ensure a proper fit between all parties. For example, in selecting a consultant, organizations should do the following:

- Identify why a consultant may be needed.

- Check to see if all internal resources have been fully tapped, and if there is an employee or someone on your staff who may be able to solve the problem.

- Solicit bids from several consultants.

- Check with colleagues for referrals and don't neglect local colleges and universities.

- Develop a list of criteria to use in judging all bidders? Common criteria include fees, on-site availability, years of experience, type of clientele served, specialties, opinions of references, and the ability to customize services.

- Thoroughly interview the top candidate(s) and solicit feedback from all staff members.

- Obtain a sample contract from the top candidates to see how they conceive the type of the

services requested within a designated timeframe.

- Consider the pros and cons of paying a flat project fee vs. an hourly fee. Avoid consultants who ask to be paid upfront or do not agree to negotiate a specific number of hours.

OUTSOURCING

One of the fastest-growing movements influencing today's WHP landscape is outsourcing. A survey of 927 companies conducted by The Wyatt Company indicates that nearly one-third of employers outsource some or all of the administration of their human resources and benefits programs. In most situations, outsourcing is referred to as a "contract service" or "vendor contract." Since the late 1980s, many employers have outsourced their health promotion operations in order to efficiently downsize, focus on their core businesses, and improve their profit margins. For a sampling of health promotion and facility management services provided by outside vendors, see table below.

Since there are no nationally recognized guidelines to use in selecting community resources, it is important to screen providers, especially those that sell products or services in the following areas: body

---

COMMONLY OUTSOURCED HEALTH PROMOTION AND FACILITY MANAGEMENT SERVICES

Health Promotion Services	**Facility Management**
• Employee health screening	• Pre-opening promotions and publicity
• Health promotion seminars	• Conducting a grand opening special event
• Health fairs	• Hiring, training, and placing fitness staff members
• Toll-free self-care services	• Establishing computerized entry and exit system
• Health promotion/benefits integration	• Conduct comprehensive pre-participation fitness evaluations
• Health awareness programs	• Supervising all exercise activities
• Health information classes	• Conducting recreational programs and leagues
• Newsletter	• Conducting on-site health fairs
• Health risk appraisals	• Implementing customized incentive programs

fat testing, employee assistance program (EAP), pre-exercise stress testing, nutritional analysis, weight management, smoking cessation, and stress management. Here are some suggested questions to ask in assessing qualifications:

1. What types of resources (personnel, money, equipment, and facilities) does the provider have to serve the company's needs?

2. Is the provider certified by a professional association?

3. Does the provider have a program or service that appears to be philosophically sound and easily understood? Are written goals, objectives, and policies clearly presented?

4. Does the provider have a clearly defined fee schedule? Is it willing to offer discounts to firms with small or no budgets?

5. Does the provider demonstrate substantial expertise in the area? Can it provide a listing of past and current clients?

6. Is the provider willing to provide a complimentary demonstration of the product or service?

7. Can products and services be customized to fit particular needs?

8. Does the provider maintain records on participants?

9. Does the provider have a formal process to evaluate their performance?

COMMERCIAL HEALTH PROMOTION MATERIALS

In the past decade, many employers have cut their workforces and, thereby, created greater workloads for fewer people. Naturally, this downsizing has created greater pressure on many organizations to stay competitive with fewer human resources. In response, more organizations are providing their health promotion staffs with health promotion kits, guides, and newsletters to better meet their programming needs. You need to examine both the situations in which you might use such materials and the materials themselves.

APPROPRIATE SITUATIONS FOR USING COMMERCIAL MATERIALS

Some of the more common arrangements in which these resources are used include the following:

• Large organizations purchasing multiple copies of resources to use in hard-to-reach locations or as stand-alone programs where there is no full-time health promotion staff. Multisite operations may have a designated employee at each site acting as a health promotion facilitator to distribute health promotion resources and motivate co-workers to promote their personal health.

• Small businesses subscribing to multimedia program kits that a designated employee (or outside vendor) can implement on a part-time basis (e.g., take-home videos supplemented with on-the-job stretch breaks).

• Health care provider organizations (managed care organizations, hospitals, clinics, and public health departments, for example) conducting actual or adapted versions of these programs at client worksites.

More employers are negotiating arrangements with managed care organizations to mail health promotion resources to employees and their dependents. In many instances, employers rely upon their managed care plan to provide health promotion and preventive care services. In one nationwide survey conducted for the Center for Corporate Health, nearly all (93 percent) of the HMOs offered members a health newsletter and/or to provide telephone-based advice services. Other activities offered by the HMOs include patient counseling and education programs (58 percent); special prenatal or maternity education programs or materials (81 percent); and self-care books dealing with prevention of or advice on common conditions and complaints to help the individual decide whether to seek medical treatment from a professional or to treat the problem at home (43 percent).

TYPES OF MATERIAL AVAILABLE

Whether an organization is starting a new WHP program or looking for ways to enhance an existing one, it is important to shop around to ensure that the resources selected can be tailored to a particular worksite. For example, assess your target population's needs and interests before purchasing a particular kit or program that may or may not meet your goals and objectives. While some programs are limited to a single topic such as exercise or back health, other programs may provide several topic-specific kits including an array of resources such as those listed here:

- Bimonthly 5- to 10-minute educational videos for employees and dependents to view at work and/or at home.

- An announcement memo sent to employees.

- A suggested time line for conducting activities.

- A ready-to-use article for the company newsletter.

- Reproducible table tents (folded index cards containing brief health messages placed on cafeteria tables).

- Large two-color program announcement posters.

- Small program announcement display posters.

- Reproducible handouts and quizzes to motivate employees.

- Facilitator guide explaining how to incorporate each kit within a suggested timeframe.

- Bimonthly facilitator newsletters.

- Participant and program evaluation forms.

CHOOSING COMMUNICATION RESOURCES

In today's fast-paced, multimedia-oriented world, a wide variety of communication resources is available to WHP personnel. Table 7.3 lists health education resources to inform, educate, motivate, and support employees in their quest for good health. Your choice of tools from this chart depends on a number of variables, including your target group's needs and interests, access to services, learning style, program goals and objectives, resources and budget, and an analysis of which tools are likely to achieve the greatest return on your investment. Learning style is particularly important to consider in selecting communication resources since people learn in different ways. Thus, various communication tools should be used to reach as many people as possible.

When reviewing the table, avoid the temptation to select only one or two tools that the table indicates will achieve a certain goal. Remember, the most cost-effective health promotion programs combine tools to achieve definable results that, when implemented, result in a cohesive intervention strategy, designed to support individual health decisions.

There are hundreds of vendors that sell commercialized WHP program materials throughout the United States. A sample listing of these vendors appears in appendix A.

This chapter has presented an overview of resources to consider in planning, implementing, and evaluating a WHP program. As the makeup of American worksites continues to change, more organizations are becoming more decentralized with multisite and culturally diverse workforces. The ability to tailor programs and resources to meet each organization's everchanging needs may well separate successful worksite programs from unsuccessful programs as we move into the 21st century.

Table 7.3 Examples of Health Promotion Communication Tools

Products and services	Communication goals						
	Generate awareness	Increase knowledge	Teach skills	Motivate change	Reinforce behavior	Support behavior	Cost per employee
Articles	3	3	1	2	2	1	*
Audiotapes	1	3	3	3	3	2	$3–$12
Books and work-books	2	3	3	2	2	1	$4.25–$12
Booklets	2	3	3	2	2	1	$1.50–$3.75
Brochures	3	3	2	2	3	1	.65–$2
Calendars	3	1	1	2	2	1	$3–$9
CD-ROM	1	3	3	3	3	1	$19–$69
Computer programs	1	3	3	2	2	1	$35–$400
Group education programs	1	3	3	3	3	3	$0–$140
Health-risk appraisal	3	2	2	3	2	2	$2.50–$18
Incentives	1	2	3	3	3	2	Donations or $
Interactive video-discs	1	3	2	3	3	1	$400–$600 per application
Magazines and journals	3	3	3	3	3	1	$1.50–$2.50 per issue
Memos	2	3	1	3	2	1	*
Newsletters	3	2	2	2	3	2	.20–.50 per issue
On-line information	2	3	2	2	2	3	$10 per hr
One-on-one counseling	1	3	3	3	3	3	$0–$125 per hr
Payroll stuffers	3	1	1	2	3	1	.15–.50
Postcards	3	1	1	2	3	1	.15–.50
Posters	3	1	1	2	3	1	$1.50–$6.00
Self-help and support groups	1	3	3	3	3	3	$0
Tabletop displays	3	2	1	2	3	1	.50–$1.50
Telephone-based services	1	3	3	3	3	3	$0–$25
Videotapes	2	3	3	3	3	1	$5–$250

Rating: 1 = low impact on communication goals; 2 = average impact on communication goals; 3 = high impact on communication goals

*Staff generated

Source: Elin Silveous and George Pfeiffer, AWHP's Worksite Health, Winter 1995. Used with permission.

CHAPTER

8

MODEL WORKSITE HEALTH PROGRAMS

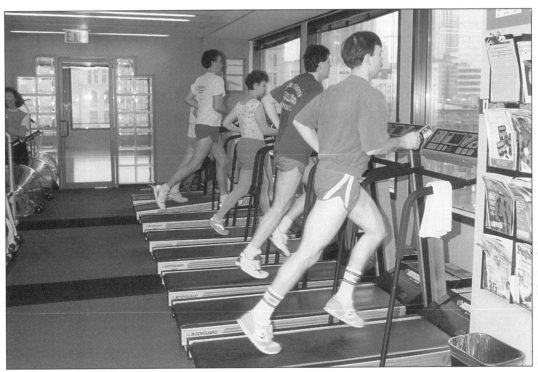

Photo courtesy of Quaker Oats

While no consensus yet exists on what comprises a model worksite health promotion program, experts agree on four prime areas of concern that WHP should address.

1. Helping employees to deal with common health problems, including stress, low back pain or injury, poor nutrition, smoking, substance abuse, weight control, poor physical fitness, lack of physical activity, and AIDS/HIV risks.

2. Promoting awareness of preventive measures such as immunization; prenatal education; and screenings, monitoring, and follow-up services for cancer, diabetes, high blood pressure, heart disease, glaucoma, and other conditions.

3. Educating employees in safety promotion and accident prevention measures, such as CPR, choke-saving techniques, emergency first aid, on-the-job safety instruction, seat-belt use, and "right-to-know"

programs on hazardous substances on and off the worksite.

4. Providing counseling services in stress management, substance abuse, drunk driving, domestic problems, financial problems, elder care, and pre-retirement planning.

MODEL WHP HEALTH PROGRAMS

Earlier in the text (chapters 3 and 4) we discussed the basic values and goals of worksite health promotion (for review, see Standards for Success, below). In this chapter we'll focus on existing programs that have had great success in meeting these goals. If you are a program planner, as you read about the strategies below, think about ways the activities might be modified to suit the circumstances at your company. If you're a student, think about and discuss the strategies that have led to success for specific programs; explore ways to apply the strategies to smaller worksites with budgeting restraints and limited resources.

THE INSIDE TRACK TOWARD HEALTH PROMOTION

When it comes to meeting employee health needs in multiple worksites, Union Pacific Railroad has given a new meaning to the term, "fitness track." UP has converted several train cars into traveling fitness centers for its "steel gangs"—workers who live in train cars for weeks at a time and make track repairs throughout the company's 21-state area. Inside the railcars, employees use both strength and aerobic equipment (multiunit weight stations, stationary bikes, rowers, dumbbells, and a heavy punching bag) and enjoy easy access to health-related literature, videotapes, and lifestyle assessment tools that help them set personal health improvement goals.

Perhaps one of the most significant accomplishments of Union Pacific's corporate-wide effort is its integrated health management system. According to the director of UP's health promotion department, "Integrating our health promotion program into our Disability Management Department has

---

STANDARDS FOR SUCCESS

What a WHP program needs . . .

Commitment from senior management to dedicate sufficient resources—funding, personnel time, equipment, and facilities. Ideally, management also shows support by participating in the program.

A clear statement of philosophy, purpose, and goals that declares the organization's commitment to motivate and assist a significant portion of employees to practice healthier lifestyles.

A process for assessment of organizational and individual needs, risks, and costs.

Leadership from well-qualified health/fitness professionals in the program's design, implementation, and ongoing operations.

A program design that addresses the most significant health risks, specific risks within the employee population, and needs of the organization.

High-quality programs that motivate participants to achieve lasting behavior changes.

Effective marketing to achieve and maintain high participation rates.

Efficient systems for program operation and administration.

Evaluation procedures for assessing program quality and outcomes.

A system of communication for sharing program results with employees, staff, and senior management.

Source: Guidelines for Employee Health Promotion Programs. Courtesy of Human Kinetics.

been one of our most successful efforts. We have numerous joint projects underway that incorporate health and fitness into our Return-to-Work program. . . . The Medical Quality Assurance process, designed by the disability management group, has saved a significant number of physician visits and lost work days over the last 8 years."

An issue receiving increased attention in the transportation industry is fatigue. UP's health promotion department conducted a pilot study among trainworkers to help them address fatigue through lifestyle changes. Because the projected benefit-to-cost ratio for this program is $3.23 to $1, UP's top management approved continuing it as well as funding other initiatives to manage fatigue.

UP offers a variety of incentives and rewards to generate and maintain employee participation. For example, employees and spouses can earn "well-bucks" for healthy behaviors. They can then use the wellbucks to purchase workout suits, water bottles, bike helmets, fire alarms, and much more.

Through innovative and consistent efforts, Union Pacific has won many awards, including C. Everett Koop National Health Awards in 1994 and 1997.

The preceding information was provided by Union Pacific Railroad. For more information on their fine WHP programs, contact Union Pacific Railroad, Department of Health Promotion, 1416 Dodge Street, Room 101, Omaha, NE 68179-0101.

Standing Guard for WHP

 Sentry

Established in 1904, Sentry has its home office in Stevens Point, Wisconsin. Sentry has 4,500 employees nationwide, with 1,700 at their home office and 600 at two other Stevens Point locations.

Sentry's health promotion and wellness programs focus on personal lifestyle choices. Sentry's wellness philosophy, as recorded in its employee handbook, reads this way:

Sentry has a strong commitment to employee wellness. Employees and their families are encouraged to participate in wellness activities. Each individual is encouraged to accept personal responsibility for his or her health and well-being. On a continuing basis the company strives to increase employee knowledge of the personal benefits derived from a well-balanced lifestyle. We believe wellness/fitness/ health promotion will help our company develop a positive mental attitude, improve productivity, reduce turnover, reduce illness, reduce health care cost, and nurture an environment conducive to personal, family, and corporate well-being.

The responsibility for the overall philosophy, direction, and implementation of wellness programming at Sentry rests with the Corporate Manager of Employee Wellness. The Wellness Department is separate from the Health Services Department. The two departments work cooperatively on various health promotion projects. The primary role of Health Services is to focus on occupational health. The department has two occupational health nurses plus support staff. Health Services administers the employee assistance program (EAP), the mandatory drug testing program, immunization clinics, glaucoma screening, blood pressure screening, stop smoking "pay back" program, and other clinical programs in addition to ensuring that Sentry meets federal requirements for occupational health. The Corporate Manager of Employee Wellness reports to the Director of Education and Training. Classes in stress management and time management are taught by the Corporate Manager of Employee Wellness. Employees may attend stress- and time-management classes on company time, but participation in exercise or wellness classes is on personal time.

Sentry's fitness program evolved from exercise sessions that began in a large coal bunker in 1961. A group of Sentry employees and townspeople, each paying a $9 lifetime membership fee, formed the "Bunker Health Club." They equipped the bunker with barbells, exercise mats, chest pulls, and other apparatus. To help employees manage stress, they converted an unused area of the bunker into a "quiet room" equipped with sofas, soft lights, and soothing music. As reflected in Sentry's wellness philosophy, WHP classes are designed to promote self-responsibility and self-empowerment.

At its central site, Sentry offers fitness, health education, recreational/social, and aquatic programs within a panorama of outstanding facilities, including a large gymnasium; a 25-meter swimming pool; two racquetball courts; two classrooms; locker rooms with showers; saunas and laundry service; and a fitness laboratory.

The fitness center is open at no cost to all Sentry employees, spouses, and dependents plus retirees and their spouses. A nominal fee is charged to participate in exercise classes such as swim lessons, aerobics, etc. The company pays about 90 to 95 percent of the costs for the physical fitness center.

The above information has been provided by Sentry Insurance. For more details on Sentry's fine program, write the Corporate Manager, Employee Wellness, Sentry Insurance, 1800 N. Point Drive, Stevens Point, WI 54481.

A Focus on Healthy Lifestyles

Public Service Enterprise Group is a publicly traded diversified energy and energy services company (NYSE: PEG) with two main subsidiaries: public Service Electric and Gas Company (PSE&G) and Enterprise Diversified Holdings, Inc. (EDHI). PSE&G is New Jersey's oldest and largest regulated utility, serving nearly three quarters of the state's population. It is one of the top ten largest combined electric and gas companies in the nation. EDHI operates Enterprise's unregulated businesses, seeking to position the company to maintain and expand its energy leadership in the region and worldwide.

Since 1991 a Comprehensive Health Awareness and Maintenance Program (CHAMP) has been offered to PSEG's 11,000 employees throughout New Jersey. In the mid '90s the program answered the challenge many programs have faced in budget and employee downsizing by initiating a process/model to redefine its mission and program model within a changing work environment. This process acknowledged the importance of linking program goals to PSEG business objectives; educating employees regarding health behavior change, self-care, and injury and disease prevention; and the systematic evaluation of various program components. The program re-engineering project was aided by several stakeholder groups used to help develop a clear direction and vision for the program.

Employee focus groups at various worksite locations provided access to employee needs, interests, and attitudes concerning health. Union and company leadership groups also provided insight into employee and company health-related issues. Steering committees at each worksite were initiated to ensure ongoing employee feedback and strengthen employee ownership. A management team representing Benefits, Safety, and Occupational Health, EAP, Disability Management, and Medical departments was formed as the Health Promotion Advisory Council (HPAC). Its major function has been to provide an integrated approach to health promotion programming by increasing the opportunity for measurable health and economic results. MediFit Corporate Services was contracted for fitness facility management and to guide the health promotion process.

The mission statement for CHAMP is to facilitate the delivery of integrated programs that support and maximize the health, quality of life, and well-being of employees. Key strategies were initiated during the re-engineering phase designed to transform the culture to support and improve health and quality of life, maximize performance and productivity, develop a strong creditable infrastructure to support the program, increase participation in program initiatives, and strengthen the communica-tion and marketing efforts. A 15-month program roll-out calendar was developed that serves as a management tool to ensure that the re-engineering goals and objectives are met. The PSEG re-engineering process/model has not only redefined the program in a rapidly changing work environment but has also been successful in renewing employee interest and participation in health and wellness.

This information was provided by PSEG and is used here with their permission. For further information on PSEG's health promotion initiatives, contact Kathleen Kostecki, Benefits Manager, at (973) 430-6064 or Laurie Jones, RD, Health Promotion Manager, at (973) 430-7918. PSEG's address is 80 Park Plaza, Newark, NJ 07102.

A Sampling of WHP Activities at Other Major Companies

Excellent WHP programs can be found throughout the United States. Here are some WHP highlights from major U.S. companies.

- **Aetna**—This employer boasts five state-of-the-art fitness centers with 7,600 enrollees and has found that its exercising employees cost $282 less per year than non-exercising employees.

- **L.L. Bean**—The Freeport, Maine-based company offers a fitness center and health promotion courses for employees. Its cholesterol-reduction program is nationally known. The program features outdoor activities such as canoeing, kayaking, and cross-country skiing. Bean pays up to $200 to employees whose families quit smoking or take prenatal classes. The payoff: per capita health insurance premiums are $2,000—half the national average.

- **Bonnie Bell**—This Lakewood, Ohio, company has a jogging path through the woods with exercise stations en route, exercise classes three times weekly, tennis courts and lessons, exercise rooms, and shower facilities.

- **Coors**—The company renovated an old grocery store into its 23,000-square-foot, state-of-the-art wellness center. Coors pays bonuses of up to $500 per family for healthy lifestyles.

- **Dow Chemical**—In 1991 this Midland, Michigan-based company completed its 23,000-square-foot Up With Life center. Nearly 19,000 square feet are used for fitness facilities such as an indoor track, cardiovascular and strength-training equipment, two aerobics studios, and men's and women's locker rooms. The remaining footage contains the health services area for health education classrooms and various clinical personnel. Dow's Backs in Action program encourages exercise, dieting, and ergonomics, which contributed to a 90% drop in on-the-job strains and sprains within 3 years.

- **First Chicago Bank**—Serving a largely female workforce, this Chicago employer pays for about 800 newborn deliveries a year. The company's wellness programs include coaching pregnant women on childbirth and giving lactating mothers a place at work to collect milk for their babies.

- **General Dynamics**—This San Diego company started its recreation program in 1949 and since then has established a wide variety of health promotion and fitness-oriented programs and facilities. Nearly 20 percent of the workers participate in the health promotion program, while close to 100 percent participate in recreation activities. The program is funded largely by on-site vending machine receipts.

- **General Electric**—GE's aircraft engine plant in Cincinnati established its fitness center in 1985, with two aerobics studios, 60 cardiovascular machines, four lines of strength-training equipment, a six-lane indoor track, an indoor pool, and classrooms. Its fine programs earned the company the Health Action Leadership Award for having the most outstanding worksite health promotion program in 1990 from Kelly Communications.

- **Mesa Limited**—Chief Executive T. Boone Pickens built a $2.5 million on-site fitness center in 1979 and established health promotion programs for Amarillo-based employees. The fitness center cuts $200,000 from the company's yearly health insurance premium.

- **Nissan Motors**—The company instills some Japanese flavor by having its Smyrna, Tennessee, employees engage in 5 minutes of group calisthenics before hitting the assembly line. Basketball goals and table tennis facilities provide exercise during work breaks.

- **Steelcase**—This company in Grand Rapids, Michigan, is known for its extensive testing of 4,000 employees for various health risks. Through risk-based programming, it expects to save $20 million in the next 10 years.

A CHAMPION FOR THE WHP CAUSE

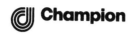

Champion International Corporation is an international paper and forest products company with 13 major facilities and nearly 200 locations in the United States. The worldwide workforce of 25,000 is primarily blue-collar workers in mostly rural locations. The company's corporate headquarters is in Stamford, Connecticut.

The first Champion fitness center opened at corporate headquarters in March 1981. By 1988 Champion had opened fitness centers in five other major locations. At all other locations it expanded the health promotion menu to include programs such as health education, medical self-care, health risk assessment, and on-site preventive services. Many of these programs are now offered to employees, dependents, and retirees.

Merging separate business departments, functions, and programs into a single, comprehensive health and family services operation is increasingly appealing to many companies, including Champion. In 1995, the company united three functions—health and fitness, employee assistance, and preventive care—into one department called Health and Family Services. To date, the results of this integration are encouraging.

Decreasing injuries and workers' compensation claims demonstrate the effect of Champion's WHP efforts on the bottom line. Other services that provide quantitative as well as qualitative data for a compelling story are the prenatal program and the preventive care plan. Says a Champion spokeswoman,

> *More often than not we talk in terms of services instead of programs, and in all communications and marketing materials, we don't forget to talk about why we offer a particular service. As a result of this integration, we see opportunities for decreasing overall operating costs and increasing support to get the resources we request. We are establishing ourselves as contributors to Champion's goals by aligning what we do with the company's goals of increased productivity and profit.*

This information has been provided by Champion International Corporation. For more details on its programs, contact the Director of Health and Family Services, Champion International Corporation, One Champion Plaza, Stamford, CT 06921.

A MODEL OF COST AVOIDANCE

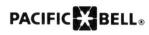

The primary rationale for WHP in the Pacific Bell program is "to develop an integrated health promotion approach involving educational, organizational, and environmental changes to improve employees' health, capabilities, and quality of worklife and to build ongoing programs that inform and motivate employees and families to adopt and sustain positive health behavior."

Full-time program staff consists of a health promotion manager, supervising exercise physiologist, staff exercise physiologist, health promotion specialist, wellness program administrator, and associates. Part-time personnel include a medical doctor, dietitian, physical therapist, cardiologist, aerobic instructors, and an additional exercise physiologist.

Programs available to employees include prenatal care, smoking cessation, back care, family care, sleep education, weight loss, cancer screening, osteoporosis screening, stress reduction, workplace violence prevention, medical consumer information, return to work, coronary risk modification, physical abilities testing, substance abuse counseling, self-care education, and weight loss.

Programs available to dependents include medical consumerism, smoking cessation, prenatal care, and weight loss. Retirees can participate in stress reduction, medical consumerism, smoking-cessation, and weight loss programs, and use the fitness facilities.

Health promotion is integrated into health benefits and involve enhanced health promotion performance standards, HEDIS (Health Plan Employer Data and Information Set) standards, expanded immunization, mammography and PAP tests, annual physicals, asthma management, smoking cessation, well baby care, and a community exercise program.

Pacific Bell has experienced measurable economic benefits from Health Promotion programs. In a recent year, cost-avoidance savings were $5,800,000, a 2.15:1 return on investment (ROI). The greatest savings were due to reduced absenteeism; employees participating in FitWorks programs (n = 8,986) were absent 3 fewer days each than employees in a matched control group. In the previous year, $4,600,000 in cost avoidance savings were reported with a ROI of 1.48.

Two efficacy studies that typify program evaluations are Breast Health and Work Hardening. The Breast Health study measured participants' health education retention and behavioral influences for breast self-examination (BSE) practices and mammography. Nearly 500 program participants were surveyed over 6 months following BSE education and mammography and were compared to a control group. Thirty-five percent of the test group compared to 22 percent of the control group stated that they practiced BSE 3 to 5 times during the previous 6 months. In addition to identifying BSE patterns, the evaluation determined that convenience was the number one reason employees participated in on-premise mammography. Work Hardening, a yearlong study of self-paced exercise programs in remote locations showed positive changes in participants' resting heart rate, blood pressure, and muscle endurance. Pacific Bell's progress earned a C. Everett Koop award in 1995.

The preceding information was provided by Pacific Bell Corporation. For more information on its WHP program, contact the Health Promotion Manager, 2600 Camino Ramon, Room 2W050E, San Ramon, CA 94589.

LIVE WELL— BE WELL

Companies of all sizes benefit from an integrated health management approach, especially larger organizations. Figure 8.1 illustrates the integration of health promotion with employee benefits at The Quaker Oats Company. The company has approximately 17,000 employees nationwide with corporate headquarters in Chicago, Illinois. The Quaker Tower's program is comprised of five uniquely separate, yet related components.

• The Fitness Center: provides the opportunity to improve flexibility, strength, endurance, and cardiovascular fitness through exercise, as well as individual lifestyle counseling regarding nutrition, weight, and stress management.

• Health Services: prevents and/or detects health risks by assisting individuals in making positive lifestyle changes that promote health and minimize illness.

• Employee Assistance Program (EAP): assists employees and eligible family members in finding alternatives for dealing with personal problems.

• Health Resource Center: promotes self-learning and supports the concept that employees can make a difference in managing their own health.

• Mothers' Room: eases the transition of returning to work for new mothers who choose to continue breast-feeding their infants.

According to the director of employee benefits,

The company's medical care costs nearly tripled between 1971 and 1981, with Quaker experiencing a 56 percent increase [from 1979–1981]. Within months we instituted a series of cost-control strategies in an attempt to slow future cost increases. Overall, I think our cost-control success is due to three major components. First, our Health Incentive Plan (HIP) give[s] employees a bigger financial stake in the cost and utilization of their medical benefits. To date, it has contributed significantly to lower health costs. Second, the Informed Choices program has helped employees and dependents understand their health care options and empowered them with cost, provider, and quality-oriented information to help them make responsible health care decisions. Third, Quaker is counting on health improvement to reduce medical cost increases in the long run as well as decrease disability claims and increase employee productivity.

The company's health promotion program, called "Live Well—Be Well," includes

• health risk appraisals and feedback through questionnaires and clinical screenings;

• behavior modification programs in areas such as nutrition, exercise, stress management, substance abuse prevention, smoking cessation, and disease management; and

- conversion of on-site nurses' clinics to more comprehensive health resource centers to assist employees on a wide range of physical and mental health matters.

Although Quaker has offered health promotion programs to employees at some locations for many years, the renewed emphasis formally incorporated the concept into its health management strategy for all areas of the company.

All Live Well—Be Well programs are free to employees, spouses, and retirees. Employees pay $10 a month to use the fitness center at the corporate facility. Other Quaker facilities with on-site centers have various arrangements from free membership to nominal fees.

Quaker provides financial incentives (up to $500 per family annually) within its flexible benefit plan to employees and spouses who meet any of eight healthy-lifestyle criteria. Employees and spouses may earn up to $140 each for making the following lifestyle pledges:

- At least 20 minutes of aerobic exercise at least 3 times a week

- Use of seat belts and car seats when driving and helmets when riding a motorcycle or bicycle

- Not to drink alcohol to excess, use illegal drugs, or misuse prescription drugs

- No use of tobacco products in the prior 6 months and a pledge not to use them in the future

Employees and spouses may also earn up to $110 each for completing a health risk appraisal, including screening for blood pressure, cholesterol, and weight. Participants' risk factors must be within guidelines, or else they must document personal efforts to reduce out-of-guideline health risk indicators, in order to receive full financial credit for the HRA screening.

In 1995, Quaker Oats earned the prestigious Well Workplace GOLD award from the Wellness Council of America (WELCOA) in recognition of its exemplary health management efforts.

This information was provided by The Quaker Oats Company. For further details about Quaker's WHP programs, contact the Manager of Benefit Plans, The Quaker Oats Company, P.O. Box 049001, Chicago, IL, 60604-9001.

A MULTISTRATEGY PFP

SAS Institute is committed to providing programs that encourage employee creativity, productivity, and loyalty. Management believes that employee

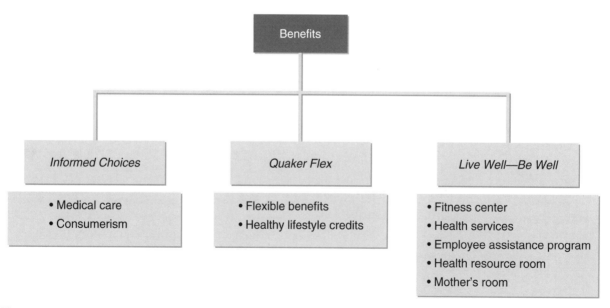

Figure 8.1 The integrated health management framework at The Quaker Oats Company.

health can be improved by offering them and their families excellent facilities and programs for fitness, wellness, and recreation.

Programs offered at SAS include aerobics (beginning, prenatal, and sports conditioning), rehabilitation programs, circuit training, racquetball, basketball, volleyball, walleyball, softball, flag football, Frisbee, table tennis, and billiards. Seminars are available on childcare, women's health, ergonomics, stress management, and smoking cessation.

A 26,000 square-foot multipurpose facility houses three racquetball courts, two basketball courts, a large exercise room, a large recreation area, a weight training room with 22 Nautilus stations, two StairMaster step machines, three Concept Two rowers, five exercise bikes, and free weights. Outdoor facilities include three lighted tennis courts, a softball field, a 2-mile running trail, and several walking trails.

This information was provided by SAS Institute, Inc. For more details about SAS Institute's program, contact Recreation and Fitness Manage SAS Institute, Inc., Box 8000, Cary, NC 27512-5000

ness memberships, and schedules and leads aerobic/fitness classes.

Healthworks facilities include several classrooms and a 3,500 square-foot fitness center with Marquette treadmills, Schwinn Air Dynes, Monarch ergometers/bikes, Avita rowers, stairclimbers, upright and semi-recumbent Life Cycles, a UBE armcrank ergometer, a cross-country skier, a Uniflex 12-station circuit trainer, a walking track, a dumbbell weight rack, and dressing rooms with lockers and showers.

Ongoing programs include cardiac rehabilitation; "Safeway to Fitness"; general fitness; weight management for adults, children and adolescents; cholesterol and blood screening; and "Heartmates" support group. Periodical programs include cholesterol treatment, worksite health screenings, smoking cessation, stress management, consulting services to business and industry, and corporate health promotion for local business.

For more information on Healthworks, contact the manager at Healthworks, Wake Medical Center, 3000 New Bern Avenue, Raleigh, NC 27610

A MODEL OF EFFICIENT USE OF SPACE

Healthworks is a division of Wake Medical Center in Raleigh, North Carolina. It is primarily a cardiovascular disease prevention program within the Wake Heart Center at Wake Medical. Healthworks' staff consists of several professionals, most with allied health backgrounds. The program manager directs the administrative and personnel operations and works directly with corporate clients. The cardiac rehabilitation nurse supervises patients, maintains charts, and recruits for the program. The cardiovascular teaching nurse teaches risk factor reduction, supervises patients, and directs much of the patient education. The registered dietitian conducts diet evaluations, consultations, and teaches weight loss classes. The exercise specialist writes exercise prescriptions, conducts fitness testing, and directs and follows patients through the cardiac rehabilitation process. The exercise technologist administers fitness assessments, coordinates adult fit-

A MODEL OF STAFF TEAMWORK

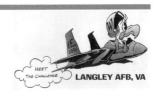

The key rationale for the Langley Air Force Base Health Promotion Program is to promote military readiness by encouraging healthy lifestyle behaviors. It is to keep its people healthy and prepared to meet the unusual requirements of the military mission.

Langley's health promotion department consists of

- a health promotion manager,

- a noncommissioned "officer in charge" and one other noncommissioned officer,

- an Installation Fitness Program Administrator,

- a dietitian,

- Nutritional Medicine Services office,

- a psychologist and a mental health clinic,

- a "Tobacco Free" program manager

- an administrator,

- a substance abuse counselor,
- a weight-management program manager,
- a "Healthy Back School" program manager,
- a cholesterol-reduction program manager, and
- the director of Managed Care.

Classes are offered to active duty members, their dependents, military retirees and their dependents, and in some instances, civilian federal employees. Frequently offered programs include:

Tobacco cessation	Healthy nutrition
Physical fitness	Back injury prevention
Cancer	Fitness assessments
Immunizations	Health risk appraisal
Cardiovascular disease prevention	Medical self-care
HIV/AIDS awareness	Alcohol and drug abuse prevention
Stress management	

The fitness center is a full-service gymnasium offering several sports competitions and activities, including racquetball, volleyball, basketball, wallyball, baseball, and football. Aerobics classes— including fitness remediation, step aerobics, and jazzercise—and martial arts classes are offered. The center holds a large and expanding weight room and an indoor lap pool. A separate aerobics equipment room offers stationary bikes, treadmills, rowing machines, recumbent bikes, and stair-steppers.

As the Air Force becomes integrated with managed care efforts, health promotion benefits are increasingly included in the provider contracts. These provider-purchased benefits include cholesterol and blood pressure screening, mammograms, health risk appraisals, and immunizations.

This information was provided by Langley Air Force Base. For more information on how Langley skillfully uses it vast array of resources as a team, contact the Health Promotion Manager, 1st Medical Group/SGPZ, 45 Pine Street, Langley Air Force Base, Virginia 23665-2080.

INTEGRATION IN A MIDSIZE WORKSITE

Lord Corporation is headquartered in Cary, North Carolina, and has three other locations; Lord's total workforce is nearly 1,600 employees. According to their manager of employee benefits,

> *. . . health and wellness programs at Lord have helped to make our employees more intelligent health care consumers, based on feedback from providers. Because we are self-insured, our health care costs vary widely from year to year with the effect of catastrophic cases. We began our cost-containment program in 1983 by reducing dental benefits, introducing managed care, initiating an ongoing and extensive communication campaign, and providing a gain-sharing incentive in which employees share cost-savings with the company.*

In 1989 Lord changed to a new in-patient hospital administrator, limited in-patient psychiatric and chiropractic benefits, set dollar limits on overall coverage, secured union agreement for direct contracting, and implemented a "defined dollar" retiree program tied to years of service. Various safety, wellness, and consumer education programs are ongoing. Overall, an integrated health management approach in which all staff members work together is the major reason for their cost-control success in the past decade. Lord's larger facilities have health promotion committees that are voluntary for employees. Management helps to design activities and programs of interest and participates in running some of the activities.

This information was provided by the Lord Corporation. For more details about Lord's WHP programs, contact the Human Resources Manager at Lord Coporation, 110 Corning Road, Cary, NC 27511.

WHP ON RELEASE TIME

ROBERT E. MASON COMPANY

The Robert E. Mason Company in Charlotte, North Carolina, has a workforce of about 100 employees. Two employees—the operations manager and the sales secretary—are given release time to administer the company's health promotion programs. Mason's Operations Manager states: "I am responsible for developing and implementing an administrative framework in which all of my official duties—ranging from health insurance benefits to the after-work fitness program—are part of an integrated network of services" (see figure 8.2).

Whether the operations manager is involved in a personnel function such as doing a new employee orientation or writing an article for the company's newsletter, she is always thinking of ways to promote the company's commitment toward employee health. For instance, how can she integrate incentives into the benefits package to motivate all employees and dependents to promote their health? Though the impact of health promotion on employee health and cost-management goals are hard to measure, Mason has more employees participating in their health fair each year and more family members are becoming involved with the program.

Mason's WHP program has resulted in lower insurance costs. Insurance premium rate increases, directly tied to employee health claims, have decreased by as much as 5 percent in some years. However, Mason has had to increase the employee deductible in some years, as well as raising each employee's out-of-pocket maximum.

Mason's WHP efforts recently earned the company its second consecutive North Carolina Governor's Council on Physical Fitness and Health Award in the small business category.

This information was provided by The Robert E. Mason Company. For more details about its WHP programs, contact the Operations Manager at The Robert E. Mason Company, P.O. Box 33424, Charlotte, NC 28233.

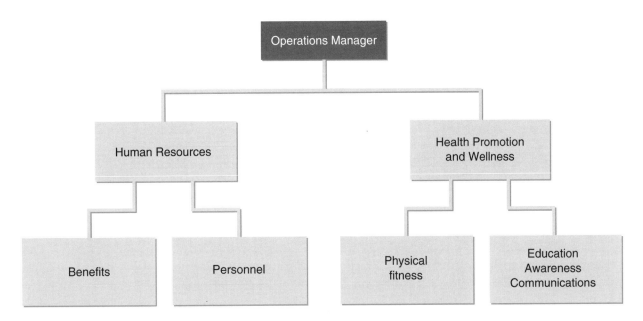

Figure 8.2 The integrated health management framework used at The Robert E. Mason Company.

What Would You Do?

Pick any one of the programs highlighted in the chapter and answer the following questions:

1. How would you adapt the program's strategies for a single-site work force of over 100 employees where management insists on a benefit-cost ratio (see chapter 5) of at least $2 to $1?

2. How would you adapt the program's strategies and activities for a worksite of 20 employees?

PART

4

OTHER CONSIDERATIONS IN WORKSITE HEALTH PROMOTION

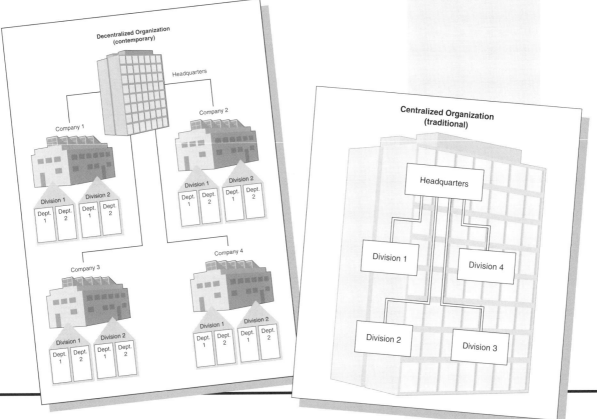

CHAPTER

9

WORKSITE HEALTH PROMOTION FOR SMALL AND MULTISITE BUSINESSES

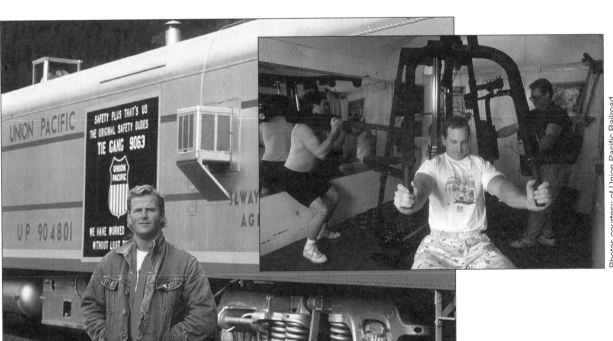

Photos courtesy of Union Pacific Railroad

Small worksites (250 employees or less) employ nearly 90 percent of the nation's workforce. The National Federation of Independent Businesses estimates that 60 percent of all businesses have fewer than 4 employees and 80 percent have fewer than 20 employees. Studies show that small businesses can benefit from WHP efforts as much as larger companies.

One of the biggest challenges facing today's health promotion personnel is to provide health promotion opportunities to all employees. With the advent of downsizing, demographic shifts, and an

127

expanding service sector, more employees find themselves working in smaller, decentralized worksites. Moreover, many of these worksites are culturally diverse and may require different strategies from those of traditional WHP programs.

In this chapter we'll discuss the challenges involved for WHP directors in planning programs that are accessible and appropriate for employees at small, multisite, and culturally diverse worksites. Although these challenges can be formidable, a sound and effective WHP strategy can almost always be developed to suit a company's circumstances.

WHP FOR SMALL BUSINESSES

Like larger employers, small businesses must minimize costs and maximize productivity to stay competitive. Containing health care costs is particularly challenging for small businesses, where even one employee's poor health might significantly damage a company's bottom line.

According to experts, the key to success for small-business WHP is management involvement. While some business owners strongly believe in employee health promotion programs, others are less enthusiastic and require evidence before they will support WHP efforts. Perhaps the best way to build the case for WHP is to show management how effective programs have been for some small businesses. Talk to program directors in your community to learn why their small-business programs succeed (or why they have failed). For a good example of a successful small-business program, see the profile on Robert E. Mason Company on page 123 in chapter 8.

WHP DISADVANTAGES AND ADVANTAGES FOR SMALL BUSINESSES

Research indicates that many small-business owners are interested in WHP activities but lack resources to plan and implement them. Obstacles to be overcome include

• **Low priority for management.** Preoccupied with productivity and cost issues, many small-business owners neglect human resource programs, including health promotion.

• **Poor financial support.** Small profit margins limit funding for programs.

• **No trained personnel.** Most smaller worksites lack employees to plan and implement WHP.

• **Lack of time.** Many small businesses operate with a minimum of workers in labor-intensive jobs with little or no flex-time.

• **Lack of facilities and equipment.** Management often feels that they cannot start something from nothing. The initial expense of equipment and modifying part of the facility for fitness and health programs often makes small-business owners view WHP as a luxury they cannot afford.

• **Low participation potential.** Smaller worksites often would have too few WHP participants to justify the resources needed for a comprehensive program.

• **No space on site.** Many small-business operations—service stations, convenience stores, fast food outlets—don't have the space to offer on-site programs.

• **Geographic dispersion.** Employees working in transportation, consulting, and sales positions are on the road much of the time, limiting their health promotion opportunities.

• **Multiple worksites.** Small numbers of employees working at several satellite locations are difficult to reach.

Despite these obstacles, small businesses have several advantages over large companies in planning WHP programs. For example, small businesses have fewer people to accommodate, which means less expense and less space to manage. Second, small businesses are often more family-oriented and close-knit than large corporations, promoting an environment that favors group participation. Third, local health agencies and organizations offering free or low-cost services often prefer to serve smaller companies. Finally, employee health improvements are more visible to co-workers, increasing the chance that others might be influenced to participate.

WHP PLANNING FOR SMALL BUSINESSES

To plan appropriate health promotion activities and programs, small businesses should follow the same procedures as larger businesses. The principles of identification, assessment, planning, implementation, and evaluation (as discussed in chapters 2 through 5) are the same regardless of the size of a business. But when a health program director plugs the unique characteristics of a small business into the general planning process, the proposal for WHP that he or she offers to management will be modified according to these characteristics. The following requirements are usually key to small-business WHP planning:

- **A flexible format.** For instance, WHP programs could be offered at the worksite or in a community center for collaborative use by several businesses.

- **Simplified equipment and space needs.** A small business does not need a large-scale workout room or enough space to accommodate a large aerobics class. Modest arrangements for employees who want to improve their health are often enough to gain significant health increases among a small work force.

- **Easy to administer.** Again, nothing fancy is required. Programs that are relatively easy to plan and implement are often sufficient at smaller companies. For example, a pre-work low back stretching and warm-up routine only requires a small area of open space and management support.

WHP programs do not have to be elaborate or expensive to be effective. In fact, most small worksite programs have no fitness facilities and require only a modest amount of money and time to administer the program. Many small businesses use community health agencies and vendors who can provide personnel, facilities, equipment, and instructional materials at little or no cost. Some of them work with sponsors such as the Chamber of Commerce, local merchant or trade associations, or shopping malls to hold events or activities.

As most small businesses have a small (or nonexistent) budget for employee health promotion programs, employee volunteers or management might use an **expense management grid** (see chapter 3, p. 39) as a guide to determine how to best use onsite and community resources. The grid can help a small business explore the feasibility of purchasing, renting, leasing, or brokering resources. For example, a rising percentage of small businesses are joining together with other small businesses to form

"pools" to negotiate purchasing products and services at discount rates. Services might include reduced employee membership fees at local health clubs, Ys, and community centers; affordable EAP services from local mental health clinics; and shared walking trails, school gymnasiums, parks, and athletic fields. As outsourcing is frequently an attractive option for small worksites, the information on outsourcing in chapter 7 (pp. 110-111) should be considered carefully by small-business health promoters.

Despite the growing success of small-business pools, many small companies might not have that option in their communities and so must resort to one-to-one arrangements with local providers. If properly structured, these arrangements can benefit both parties. For instance, the partnership between the Wisconsin-based Copps grocery store chain and the YMCA has become a model for small businesses. Copps contracted with the Y to provide a three-phase WHP program consisting of fitness testing/consultation, health education, and special recreational opportunities. Nearly half of Copps' employees participate in the program. The success of the arrangement has had widespread value, benefiting not only Copps and the Y but the entire community as other area businesses establish similar programs.

HEALTH INSURANCE COVERAGE

Nearly two-thirds of the 44 million Americans without health insurance are in families headed by a full-time worker, most working at very small businesses. The high cost of providing health insurance coverage to employees and dependents is prohibitive for many small business owners. Many employees at these businesses shop the insurance market for the best deal, often changing insurers every year. Millions of others go without health insurance, forced to risk the devastating consequences of accidents or long-term illness because they simply cannot afford to pay health insurance premiums.

Some small companies are helping their employees via health insurance pooling. A well-publicized example is a group of small businesses in Cleveland, Ohio, that formed a large pool called the Council of Smaller Enterprises (COSE). The council consists of 9,000 firms representing 54,000 employees and 120,000 dependents. All COSE members can purchase affordable health insurance coverage because the council has persuaded large insurers to offer their coalition the same advantages given to larger companies. The most important of these advantages is the clout to pressure doctors and hospitals to keep costs down. The COSE arrangement has been a successful cost-control strategy for its members, whose annual premiums typically rise only about one-fourth as much as they do for non-COSE businesses.

Lifestyle Factors

Increasingly, the availability and cost of a company's health care plan depends on employees' health risks. In such a case, a company might only be able to afford insurance that does not pay claims directly tied to a person's choice, such as smoking-induced lung diseases or injuries received during motor vehicle accidents in which safety belts were not worn. Or the company might be willing to pay the basic, low-risk rate but require that employees pay the difference if their lifestyle choices result in higher risk. In either of these cases, a primary goal of WHP would be to motivate high-risk and unhealthy employees to reduce their risk factors.

Evaluating WHP Programs in Small Businesses

Although they are not as likely as larger companies to have data-management systems for tracking absenteeism, productivity, health care use, and so on, small businesses can monitor certain types of data to evaluate health promotion efforts. Evaluation procedures that can be modified to suit small-business programs are discussed in chapter 5. At a minimum, employee participation should be tracked to evaluate interest in different types of health promotion programs. Health status indicators such as blood pressure, body fat percentage, and low back flexibility can also be easily monitored to tell program

directors and management whether particular programs are working.

In planning an evaluation, small businesses should not overlook possible assistance from local health associations and the prospects for creating collaborative arrangements. For example, faculty members at a local college may be interested in providing evaluation assistance in exchange for using a small company as a research site.

Although small businesses often need to find innovative ways to evaluate their programs, evaluation is a step that should never be neglected. A WHP program that does not evaluate itself will have no evidence that the program should be continued, greatly increasing the chances that management will consider WHP to be expendable.

WHP for Multisite Businesses

With trends continuing for businesses to place their workforce at multiple strategic or convenient locations, creating WHP programs to meet the needs of multisite companies has become a common challenge for health promoters. When working with multisite populations, program directors will need to develop programs and policies based on the combined data from *all* sites. The data collected from site to site will often vary, and the program itself may need to vary in order to meet each site's unique needs.

Organization Structure

Generally speaking, multisite businesses fall into two categories of organization: **centralized,** which is the traditional structure, and **decentralized,** a

---

Risk-Reduction Actions on a Small Scale

Even relatively minor risk-reduction actions can pay off for small businesses. Consider two employees with chronic back problems. John works for a large company with 1,000 employees, whereas Charlie works for a small company of 20 employees. From a risk-management and economic point of view, John's health care costs associated with his back problem can be spread among 999 other employees, whereas Charlie's costs are spread among only 19 other employees. Consequently, Charlie's condition increases his company's health insurance risk far more than John's condition and so makes it increasingly difficult for this company to qualify for—much less afford—today's costly health insurance coverage. Fortunately, today's health insurance "pools" (alliances) are closing this gap for many small businesses.

more contemporary structural organization. Refer to figures 9.1 and 9.2 for models of the two structures.

Multisite programming varies depending on the organizational structure. If a company is centralized, the headquarters facility generally funds and directs WHP programs to the field. The headquarters staff develops the materials and rolls out the program through field coordinators (who are generally non-health professionals). Although a company may be centralized and funded by a corporate headquarters, if the local sites are dispersed throughout the United States or abroad, cultural differences can greatly affect health promotion outcomes.

If a company is decentralized, the local site tends to have more control over WHP programming. The local sites fund programs and generally want more customization. For example, a corporate goal may be to "provide a safe and healthy work environment." The operating division may adapt this broad goal by adding specific goals, such as the following:

- Provide a back injury prevention program to reduce back injury costs by 50 percent.

- Provide healthy food options in the cafeteria.

- Encourage and help each employee to be as healthy and productive as possible.

Although a decentralized organization presents more challenges for WHP, a program director's considerations are similar for the two structures. In each case the director must find a way to modify the WHP planning framework (presented in chapter 2, p. 18) to meet the needs of a multisite operation. In the sections that follow, the major components of the framework (identification, assessment, implementation, and evaluation) will be discussed as they relate to a company with employees spread among two or more locations.

IDENTIFICATION AND ASSESSMENT

As is true at a single-site location, planning WHP for a multisite program first involves identifying and assessing employee needs and interests. When a business has employees at several hard-to-reach and/or very different types of sites, identification and assessment become particularly important phases of the process. Review chapter 2 for details about these phases. For multisite programming, the key components within the two phases are to

- visit the sites and meet with management,

- learn current policies and procedures, and

- understand the site's internal systems, e.g., operations, databases, interdepartmental communication, etc.

VISITING THE SITES AND MEETING WITH MANAGEMENT

A first step is to visit the sites and talk to key members of management. Depending on the number of locations, you may want to start with a survey to learn about employee demographics, areas of greatest needs, shift schedules, cultural diversity, and types of work performed. This survey can be mailed out ahead of your visit so that you have time to weigh the results before you meet with employees and management.

To make your site visit most effective, talk to both management and employees to get an accurate read on the site. Discuss safety issues, site morale, health concerns, health care benefits, and union representation. If possible, work an off-schedule shift (e.g., third shift on an offshore oil platform), as this is a

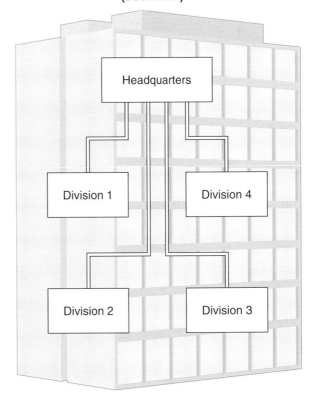

Figure 9.1 A centralized (traditional) organizational framework.

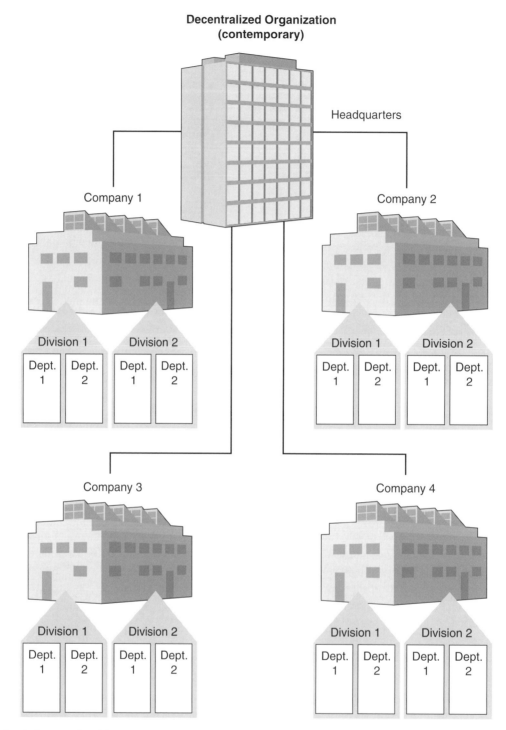

Decentralized Organization (contemporary)

Headquarters

Company 1

Division 1
| Dept. 1 | Dept. 2 |

Division 2
| Dept. 1 | Dept. 2 |

Company 2

Division 1
| Dept. 1 | Dept. 2 |

Division 2
| Dept. 1 | Dept. 2 |

Company 3

Division 1
| Dept. 1 | Dept. 2 |

Division 2
| Dept. 1 | Dept. 2 |

Company 4

Division 1
| Dept. 1 | Dept. 2 |

Division 2
| Dept. 1 | Dept. 2 |

Figure 9.2 A decentralized (contemporary) organizational framework.

good opportunity to show employees that you are there to help them, not just management.

Along with meeting employees and management, seek health care utilization and cost data reports to determine which health care facilities are most frequently used. Try to also interview health staff from other companies in the area that offer WHP.

LEARNING CURRENT POLICIES AND PROCEDURES

During your site visit, get a copy of an employee handbook or policy and procedure manual. Review the document, looking at areas that influence the health of the work environment. Learn about the site's smoking policy, flextime policy, mandated safety or illness and injury prevention programs, sick leave and family leave, cafeteria and vending machines, worksite violence prevention program, drug and alcohol screening programs, return-to-work program, pre-employment screening process, and other items pertaining to employee health and lifestyles.

UNDERSTANDING THE SITE'S INTERNAL SYSTEMS

Understanding the site's organization allows for more comprehensive WHP planning. The better you develop your programs to align with current organizational systems, the more likely the programs will succeed. During your site visit, talk to human resource personnel to learn how to make changes in policy. If there is an employee union, also try to understand the union/management relationship and the process used to reach consensus. Other internal systems to inquire about include safety practices, medical management, communication systems, hiring and training practices, and total quality-management practices.

IMPLEMENTATION

Refer to chapter 4 to review general guidelines for implementing WHP programs. Additional steps involved in implementing programs specifically for multisite businesses include recruiting volunteer coordinators; considering the addition of staff to reach all sites; rewriting internal policies and procedures; following up on communication with management, employees, volunteers, and any WHP staff; developing programs to encourage self-responsibility; considering readiness to change; targeting high-risk employees; emphasizing self-care programs; and weighing other critical considerations. Each of these steps will be discussed in detail in the sections that follow.

RECRUITING VOLUNTEER COORDINATORS

With limited resources, most multisite programs are run by volunteer employee coordinators. It's important to provide guidelines to the site on selection of volunteer coordinators. Criteria for these guidelines should include:

- All employee coordinators should be true volunteers, not appointed volunteers
- One management representative
- One representative from each department/division

- Divide the coordinators by those most and least likely to participate
- Balance committee with cultural diversity
- Balance committee with men and women
- Balance committee with an employee from every shift
- If spouses are included, ask a spouse to participate

This volunteer committee will need ongoing support and guidance from you to ensure responsibility and focus. Having the committee develop a charter is helpful; this includes length of commitment, roles and responsibilities, and expectations of communication.

An option for the volunteer committee is to dedicate 10 to 15 hours a week of each employee's job responsibilities toward the program.

ADDING STAFF TO REACH MULTISITES

During the development and implementation of awareness and basic education programs for employees, a non-health professional can roll out and follow up with many program materials provided by you. But as the site matures and more focused education and behavior change programs are developed and implemented, the need for professional assistance arises. During the development of the program, calculate this need with number of hours, cost, and responsibilities. Staffing options vary depending on site funding and demand. Some of these options include the following:

- Providing an internship to a student from a local university
- Providing a mentorship to a local physical therapist
- Hiring a local vendor
- Hiring and training a local team of professionals to go on location assignments
- Teaming with the local health plan to provide the service at a reduced rate, or teaming with local medical providers

Internally training the individual selected will help ensure a clear understanding of overall program goals. Front load the on-site staff with the customer research data and the marketing processes to make sure they understand management's view and level of commitment so they can accommodate employees with disabilities, less education, and liability concerns. The better they fit into the cultural norms, the fewer barriers to participation.

REWRITING INTERNAL POLICIES AND PROCEDURES

For your WHP programs to work, it's critical for company policies to align with program interventions. For instance, smoking policies should support smoking-cessation efforts, the cafeteria or vending machines should provide healthy meals consistent with your nutrition and weight-management programs, employee hours need to be flexible enough to allow participation in health promotion activities, and so on. Worksite health programs that are inconsistent with overall company policies reduce the programs' credibility and practically ensure failure.

FOLLOWING UP ON COMMUNICATION

Before implementing a program, revisit the initial discussions you had with site management to ensure that the program's goals match up with management expectations.

You might put agreements in writing to reconfirm all parties' commitment to responsibilities, costs, time lines, and follow-up procedures. The more health promotion is integrated with other company functions, the greater the importance of this communication, as all parties should be involved on a regular basis. With most multisite programs the presence of a health professional is not on-site, and generally an employee's job responsibility does not include health promotion. Thus it is easily put aside without on-site presence.

DEVELOPING PROGRAMS TO ENCOURAGE SELF-RESPONSIBILITY

Most multisite programs do not have the benefit of an on-site health professional. Although all programs should encourage employee self-responsibility, multisite populations without immediate resources need to be developed and implemented with self-responsibility in mind. Plan programs with a facilitative approach rather than a direct approach. Instead of telling employees what to do to be healthy, motivate them through education about the effects of their lifestyle choices. Give them options they can tailor to meet their goals and fit their situations and values. As one doctor has put it, "We need to adopt the attitude that we may be great coaches, but we cannot ourselves get out there and win the ball game."

CONSIDERING READINESS TO CHANGE

In dispersed workforces, organization change and issues will be different—for example, one site may be in union negotiation, another may be downsizing, and still another may be undergoing an analysis for a specific problem. Given the changing variables within each organization, program implementation may look different, and timing will vary from year to year on site requests. To ensure that organizational needs are met, develop core content that can be flexible and customized to cultural demands. When assessing individual need and readiness to change, include physiological risk factors, current behavior/habits, psychological factors, and social support. Most health risk appraisals provide this type of individual assessment. Research and understand cultural predisposition to certain genetic health risks, as well as cultural lifestyle patterns; this is where the local public health department and local medical providers can be of guidance.

Review the following "readiness-to-change" model (modified from DiClemente and Proschaska):

The Process of Change in Behavior

1. **Precontemplation**—Individual is unaware, unwilling, or discouraged when changing problem behavior.

2. **Contemplation**—Individual is considering the prospects of change and researching information about the pros and cons of the change.

3. **Preparation**—Individual intends to make change in the near future; he or she has learned valuable lessons from past attempts and failures.

4. **Action**—Individual takes action to change behavior.

5. **Maintenance**—Individual attempts to sustain change and avoid relapse.

6. **Termination**—Individual does not think about and is not tempted by the past problem behavior.

By assessing and gathering baseline data on individuals, you can better develop and implement different intervention options that will appeal to people in different stages of change. Provide self-responsible options and choices from group programs to individual programs and from corporate-based to community/health plan-based programs. Understand the culture to know if tangible incentives extrinsically motivate employees to start behavior change. Rely on your volunteer committee and local resources to enhance your decisions while developing and implementing programs. Many times you will find individual readiness to change, but the organizational environment cannot support the process. This is where flexibility and knowledge as well as utilization of resources become critical.

TARGETING HIGH-RISK EMPLOYEES

Further implementation for multisite programs encourage ongoing awareness campaigns, health fairs, and group education programs. As resources remain limited, shifting delivery from untargeted, group-based health promotion to targeting the high-risk employees is proving to be the most cost-effective approach. To make the most impact, target the high-risk group that is the most ready to change.

Historically, WHP efforts have not adequately addressed "relapse," which is the greatest barrier to permanent lifestyle change. Research conducted by StayWell Health Management Systems, Inc., indicates that targeting employees with high-risk profiles who are ready to change increases the potential for long-term behavior change. High-risk employees generally require proactive, ongoing support. Note the comparison in table 9.1 of the traditional model versus the focused intervention model developed by StayWell. Focused interventions are designed specifically to identify and motivate high-risk individuals toward risk-reduction action. Thus, by shifting funds from group-based programming to a high-risk focus, you are more likely to impact your program goals sooner and sustain long-term results.

EMPHASIZING SELF-CARE PROGRAMS

Medical self-care programs assist in lowering the demand for health care by helping employees enhance their decision-making skills, improve the quality of self-care they practice, and communicate effectively with their health care providers. With

Table 9.1 A Comparison of a Traditional and a Focused Health Promotion Intervention	
Traditional intervention	**Focused intervention**
General Promotion	**Personalized Promotion**
Posters and flyers	Individualized based on interest, need, risk, and readiness
Newsletter articles	Target marketing to specific individuals
Time-based assessment	**Participation and Risk-Based Assessment**
Annual or scheduled assessments	Targeting nonparticipants
	Individuals with specific risks would increase assessments
Not based on risk, just age and sex	New preventive exam schedules will focus on risk with follow-up appropriate to risk
Untargeted Group Education	**Individually Focused Education**
Same class to all; consider need or interest	Invitation to specific risk-based class
	Target to match individual need with type of education and individual preference
	Traditional class with group program but also does not offer one-one counseling or self-study.
Reactive Maintenance (the problem of relapse is ignored or addressed only after relapse has occurred)	**Proactive Support and Follow-Up**
	Identify and build in support, counseling, and one-on-one opportunities as part of the delivery process
	Built in maintenance, appropriate follow-up, and facilitation skills
"Add-On" Evaluation	**Integrated Evaluation**
After the fact evaluation	Built-in to process prior to delivery
Unfocused metrics	Appropriate and effective measures focused on risk reduction

Courtesy of StayWell Health Management Systems, Inc.

multisite programs comes a variety of health plan models from a HMO or PPO to an indemnity plan. Some multisite programs have over 50 health benefit plans throughout the nation available to their employees.

WEIGHING OTHER
CRITICAL CONSIDERATIONS

Multisite programs differ most in the need for flexibility and creativity in implementation and delivery methods. Factors such as decentralization, site-driven funding, culturally diverse employee groups, blue- versus white-collar employees, limited staffing issues, organizational readiness, and individual readiness challenge the health professional to meet multifaceted needs at different times and in customized ways. Niche programming for the local culture is critical. Spending time in their environment, especially with blue-collar employees, cultivates trust and a relevant understanding of their job, which is extremely important to them.

EVALUATION

Considerations for multisite program evaluation are more complex than a single-site evaluation. Some issues unique to multisite evaluation are discussed in the sections that follow.

MANAGEMENT SUPPORT

Throughout the life of the program, contact with management is essential. The more decentralized the program, the more time you find yourself obtaining ongoing support and focus for the health promotion program. It is wise to have a broad base of management support and not rely on one champion at the site. For example, you may have 40 sites, with five to seven managers at each site. Of course the possibility for turnover and rotation of these managers creates an ongoing process of educating management on key issues, focus, and outcomes.

ACHIEVING GOALS AND OBJECTIVES

During the initial proposal writing and planning meetings with management, bring an evaluation plan to base decisions on. Managers who are unaware of the benefits of health promotion and preventive health services may have a difficult time determining and articulating their desired outcome. Lead them by offering options, especially in a multisite environment where decentralized managers are looking for specific goals. An effective and cost-

efficient strategy is to facilitate consensus of goals and objectives across all multisite management teams. Work with the organization's business plan and metrics and lay out the evaluation plan within the existing framework. Be realistic in your evaluation plan; with multisite reporting in the data, your process for collection must be simple. Clarify in writing the data you need from each site in order to meet its goals and objectives. For example, you need either to receive health plan utilization from human resources or you need a copy of the monthly incident report. Reach consensus with other functional groups on how this data should look when you receive the information.

PROGRAM TRACKING

Program tracking is the most critical component of a multisite program and evaluation. The need for a data-management system and clear utilization process to link the integrated program is key to evaluation success. Linking systems through a computer-wide area network, local area network, or e-mail to coordinate the multisite data collection is a good option. For very small multisite locations, you may have the volunteer committee complete a standard evaluation form to send to a centralized data collection site. In any case, the tracking system for evaluation must be clearly thought out, planned, and funded at the outset of the program.

PROGRAM EFFECTIVENESS

Program effectiveness is usually gauged by the ratio of benefit to cost. With multisite programs, you may be required to report program effectiveness by location. Suppose one of your multiple sites decides to implement a program that includes an initial survey, a health fair with HRAs and screenings, and a high-risk target follow-up for 10 percent of the site employees. How will you measure this one site's return on investment? Does the benefit-to-cost ratio fit your overall strategy to support the goals and objectives?

PARTICIPATION AND ADHERENCE

The data-tracking system should enable seamless recording of participation and adherence levels. Number of employees in attendance should be tracked, and program utilization or penetration should be calculated. Each independent site should be given feedback as well as aggregate data collected on all multiple sites. Monitor employee adherence to an activity and track behavior change. Record how many high-risk and multiple-risk

Table 9.2   A Sample Management Satisfaction Survey

Thank you in advance for sharing your input on Preventive Health Services (PHS). Your response is very important to our continuous improvement process. Since we are requesting feedback from several different perspectives at many of Chevron's worksites, we would greatly appreciate it if you would complete this survey yourself and NOT pass it on to someone else. Please return this survey by October 12 to the address on the reverse side.

I. Each statement below describes a specific aspect of Preventive Health Services (PHS). Using the following scale, please indicate how much you agree or disagree with each statement.

	Strongly disagree	Disagree	Somewhat disagree	Somewhat agree	Agree	Strongly agree
1. Our PHS Advisor has contacted me to describe the range of services PHS provides	1	2	3	4	5	6
2. PHS is an important resource because it helps my employees be more productive	1	2	3	4	5	6
3. PHS provides information that helps create/maintain a healthy workforce in order to meet our business objectives	1	2	3	4	5	6
4. My employees utilize PHS	1	2	3	4	5	6
5. Our PHS Advisor responds to our needs quickly	1	2	3	4	5	6
6. Our PHS Advisor sees goals and priorities to accomplish results	1	2	3	4	5	6
7. Our PHS Advisor demonstrates the expertise to meet our needs	1	2	3	4	5	6
8. Our PHS Advisor suggests creative solutions to address our needs	1	2	3	4	5	6
9. Our PHS Advisor works effectively with us/our employees to deliver services	1	2	3	4	5	6
10. Our PHS Advisor expresses her-/himself clearly	1	2	3	4	5	6
11. Our PHS Advisor demonstrates effective presentation skills	1	2	3	4	5	6
12. Our PHS Advisor gives us a written annual summary of services delivered	1	2	3	4	5	6
13. The services offered by PHS have been of benefit to my employees in areas such as employee safety, health, and commitment to the company and are therefore worth the cost	1	2	3	4	5	6
14. I will continue to utilize PHS	1	2	3	4	5	6

(continued)

Table 9.2 *(Continued)*

II. We have used the following Preventive Health Services (check all that apply):

____ Annual wellness program

____ Back injury prevention

____ ERT/firefighter physical conditioning

____ Fitness facility consultation

____ Health education

____ Health fair

____ Health plan coordination (regarding Preventive Services)

____ Health risk assessment and blood pressure/cholesterol screening

____ Health Quest University

____ Healthy cafeteria/vending nutritional consultation

____ Initial PHS consultation

____ Newsletter/health awareness articles

____ Office ergonomics

____ Smoking policy development and smoking-cessation programs

____ Other (please print) _____

_____

III. My primary reasons for utilizing HS are (rank from 1–5 with 1 as the most important):

____ Demonstrate commitment to employees and their health

____ Improve on-/off-job safety

____ Increase employee morale

____ Increase employee productivity

____ Reduce health-related risks

____ Support incident-free operations

____ Other: _____

_____

IV. Please tell us something about yourself.

OpCO: _____

Your work type: ____ Human Resources ____ Safety ____ Other _____

V. Comments _____

_____

Courtesy of Chevron Preventive Health Services

employees attended the program. Participation can be tracked by requesting referrals as a measurement of integration.

INTEGRATION

Planning processes are essential to the assurance of consistent development and growth of your program. As integration at each multisite heightens, the more checks and balances are needed to ensure process efficiency. Process evaluation of each functional group and the integration links are critical to maximizing outcomes and program impact. Other functional groups collect data in collaboration with one data-management system or independently (e.g., health plan utilization, safety records, and workers' compensation data). Yet the overall process of data integration impacts outcomes. The opportunity for duplication of services, costs, and low communication grows as the integration spreads without control.

CUSTOMER SATISFACTION AND EMPLOYEE COMMITMENT

Survey your multisite management customers throughout the life of the program to ensure independent satisfaction and to gather feedback. Distribution of an employee survey measuring level of commitment and behavior change opinions, questioning motivational levels, and providing the opportunity to offer feedback allows refocus and insurance for program outcome and impact. An important goal of an evaluation strategy is to provide feedback that you will continually communicate to management and employees.

Here are some of the services offered by Chevron's Preventive Health Services (PHS) to Chevron worksites worldwide:

Services	Description of services
Planning/assessment	
Annual plan	A PHS advisor discusses your business needs and describes PHS services available. A plan is made for delivery of those that involve outside vendors.
Health plan coordination	Work with Chevron health plans to evaluate preventive services and maximize their accessibility to their employees and their families. Often includes free delivery of health promotion services at the worksite.
Health risk assessment and blood pressure/cholesterol screening	Provide a health risk assessment (HRA) that uses medical screening values (blood pressure and cholesterol) and a health questionnaire to identify employee health risks. All employees receive feedback. Groups with 50+ HRAs completed receive an aggregate report of group risks. HRAs are repeated every 3 years and screenings are recommended annually.
Initial consultation	Review preventative health services business plan and cost/services. Discuss customer needs and business values.
Awareness	
Health fair	Coordinate an event where health-related vendors provide materials on a variety of health/wellness topics for the purpose of increasing participant awareness of health issues and referral sources.
Health Quest	Provide turnkey modules on health promotion topics that address health risk areas. Topics include back injury prevention and nutrition. Ideal for safety meetings.
Newsletter articles	Develop and distribute schedules of services and programs or articles within local newsletters focusing on healthy lifestyle topics. PHS provides articles on a wide range of topics.
Preventive exam	Coordinate regular reminders to all employees encouraging them to schedule preventive exams and explaining the guidelines for preventive exam content.
Healthy workplace	
Fitness center	Provide guidance on establishing supervised or unsupervised facilities with aerobic programs and cardiovascular, strength, and endurance equipment.
Facilities	Offer health and fitness programs that encourage healthy lifestyle habits.
Nutrition consultation	Provide suggestions to caterers regarding healthy choices and alternatives in menu selections. Work with customers on providing healthy choices in the vending machines.
Smoking policy	Written smoking-cessation policy exists and is communicated at the site.

(continued)

ONE CORPORATION'S APPROACH (CONTINUED)

Services	Description of services
Healthy workplace (continued)	
Back injury prevention	Train supervisors, employees, and ergonomic committees to review correct lifting mechanics, apply NIOSH guidelines to work situations, and address behavior changes to prevent injury.
ERT/firefighter physical conditioning	Train ERT and firefighters, including a physical assessment and exercise guidelines applicable to ERT duties, safe lifting techniques, and back injury prevention.
Office ergonomics	Train supervisors, employees, and employee coaches to identify correct ergonomic principles and encourage behavior change to prevent injury.
Pretask safety stretching	Implement a before-work stretching program in an effort to reduce potential injury.
Behavior change	
Healthy eating and weight control	Provide guidelines on healthy eating, such as cooking classes or weight-management programs.
Incentive program	
Consultation/development	Provide guidance on effective and appropriate incentives to motivate all employees to participate in healthy lifestyle activity.
Self-care	A comprehensive medical self-care book is offered to all employees. Use of the manual is reinforced through training and incentives.
Smoking cessation	Resources range from self-help materials to referral to group programs.

SUMMARY

Multisite program planning requires tenacious communication, clarification, and follow-up to management customers. Organizations in continually changing environments have a tendency to work as a single site in a vacuum, which creates barriers for the programmer planning multisite global processes. Critical success factors for a multisite program manager include high integration, along with reaching all levels of employees with communications and program penetration. Ensure this by working with them on their shift, in their work environment; be real and honest with these employees. Ask the customer what is wrong with the program and how it can be improved. Customers are your ultimate audience and their empowering trust to you comes only with real personal presence and experience.

What Would You Do?

Small Businesses

In your quest to find a summer job, you land a part-time sales position with a small auto parts distributor (50 employees). During your first week, the personnel director distributes a storewide memo (a) announcing the store's health care costs have increased 25% over the past year's costs, (b) that nearly 50% of the increased costs are due to low back injury claims, and (c) that all employees will have to contribute $150 more per month to maintain their health insurance benefits. As you size up the situation, the thought of proposing a pre-work low back stretching program on work time comes to mind. You assume that such a program (a) may demonstrate to the health insurer that the store is commited to reducing its low back injury risk and (b) would "buy more time" for the store to show that it can lower this risk and associated costs. With your game plan in mind, what obstacles should you consider in selling this proposal to the personnel director and eventually to the insurer to give the program a chance to reduce low back risks?

For more information on health promotion resources for small businesses, please refer to appendix A.

What Would You Do?

Multisite Businesses

Read the following descriptions of different worksites, all of which are part of the same corporation, and choose one.

Case Study #1: A coal mine in New Mexico employs 85% Navajo American Indians. Total employee population is 375 people (90% men and 10% women). The workforce is unionized and works 3 rotating 8-hour shifts. The mine has 3 different sites with separate entrances. The union participates in a nationwide health plan negotiated specifically for coal miners, which includes little preventive care. Management will only participate and pay for preventive activities if employees drive the program.

Case Study #2: A refinery in the Gulf Coast area employs 90% men and 10% women. The total employee population is 1,200, with an average age of 42. The non-union plant requires 70% blue-collar work and works 2 rotating 12-hour shifts. A health promotion program has been in place for 2 years with an on-site facility of 10,000 square feet. The top employee risk factors are poor eating habits, stress, back injuries, high blood cholesterol, and lack of exercise.

Case Study #3: In a large Midwestern city, a cellular phone company has 5 worksites with a total of 1,500 white-collar employees. The population is 50% male and 50% female, with an average age of 34. The majority of employees have a college education and the company is non-union. Access to health promotion and risk-reduction programs is limited to the choice of two managed care programs.

Case Study #4: Located on the east coast are 55 offshore oil platforms that house 15 to 40 employees at each platform bunkhouse. Each facility has a catered food arrangement and 17 of the platforms have fitness facilities. The employee population is non-union and 90 percent blue-collar males. The employees belong to a traditional indemnity (fee-for-service) plan, and emergency care is the most common claim.

After reviewing the strategies for managing multisite WHP programs described in this chapter, select one of the case study sites and create ideas for conducting each of the four activities listed below:

1. Employee research
2. Marketing
3. Development and Implementation
4. Evaluation

10

PROFESSIONALLY
PREPARING
FOR THE WORKSITE

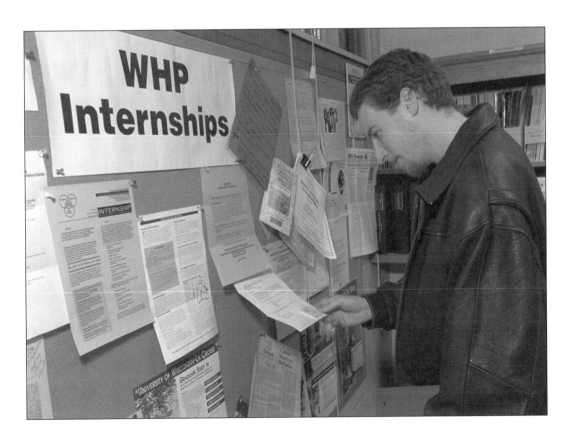

The majority of North America's large companies (more than 1,000 employees) have some type of worksite health promotion program. Many of these programs were developed in the 1970s and 1980s; some got started in the 1990s. In the late 1990s—and, by projection, into the early 2000s—as many

worksites cut their workforces, we in the field of WHP are anxious to see the impact of this downsizing. What does the future have in store for WHP? This is certainly a provocative and timely question, and one that we believe will have a satisfying response. Despite the current trend of widescale downsizing (or maybe *because* of this trend), as WHP's potential as a money saver is recognized and publicized, the more it will be embraced by its skeptics. We believe that our field has a promising future, especially for enthusiastic and energetic individuals who prepare for it!

ESSENTIAL SKILLS FOR ENTERING THE WHP FIELD

What are the essential skills for successfully entering an uncertain job market? To identify the most desirable skills for entry-level health promotion and fitness specialists, we reviewed three independent surveys. The first survey was conducted in the late 1970s and focused on competencies; the second was conducted in the 1980s and focused on recommended college courses. The findings of the third survey—involving nearly 200 WHP program directors from educational, corporate, and hospital settings—support many of the ones reported in the previous surveys. This survey, conducted by researchers at the University of Wisconsin at Stevens Point, indicates that when hiring new employees, program directors tend to value certain behaviors, knowledge, and skills (see table 10.1). Overall, the surveys reflect an increased emphasis on a broad background, especially for those hoping to become program managers or directors.

DEVELOPING STANDARDS

Since the early 1990s, the Association for Worksite Health Promotion (AWHP) has been working with other national health organizations in an industry-wide effort to develop WHP program standards that may lead to a program accreditation process. The main functions of the WHP director are divided into three broad areas: business management, program management, and human resource management. This delineation provides professionals and employers with a framework for enhancing the overall quality of WHP programs and the professionals who oversee them. For a listing of the 96 skill areas, refer to appendix C on page 165.

ACADEMIC PREPARATION

To meet the health management needs of employers, more colleges and universities are offering courses in WHP and related disciplines. Since changes occur every year, compare programs closely before committing to a particular university or major field of study. Speak with faculty members to learn about career options, specific courses, faculty experience, internship opportunities, job prospects after graduation, where past graduates are working, graduate school possibilities, and so on. Ask to see copies of course syllabi so you can evaluate the

---

Table 10.1 Behaviors, Knowledge Areas, and Skills Most Commonly Desired by Program Directors, in Order of Ranked Preference

Behaviors	Knowledge areas	Skills
Shows initiative	Behavior change	Motivating participants
Models a healthy lifestyle	Physical health	Giving presentations
Demonstrates team attitude	Stress management	Assessing fitness
Sensitive to diversity	Nutrition	Health counseling
Does more than job requires	Aerobic exercise	Assessing and interpreting health data
Respects company	Emotional health	Marketing programs
	Health care cost control	Leading behavior change groups
	Utilizing health care systems	Designing incentive programs
		Using health care policy and procedures data to plan programs

topics covered in each course. Review this information and talk with a faculty member to determine if a particular academic program really reflects today's marketplace and your career interests. If possible, select a program that centers on but is not limited to health promotion. A good academic program includes a mixture of specialty and generic courses, as well as practice or an internship in a real work setting.

To succeed in today's competitive marketplace, you'll need a strong base of skills in health promotion, exercise science, and business management. A multifaceted background will be particularly important as career options evolve and companies look for one person to play multiple roles. Versatility can be the crucial ingredient for moving into an advanced position.

PUTTING YOUR PROGRAM TOGETHER

Among the tips for preparing for a career in health promotion is to avoid the easy courses that so many students are tempted to take. Yes, these courses can boost your GPA, but they won't win you many points in the job market. Today's marketplace is increasingly competitive; prepare for what's ahead by making your curriculum competitive, too. The following are among the upper-level courses you should consider taking:

- Health Promotion
- Anatomy and Physiology
- Health Behavior
- Health Problems
- Injury/Accident Control
- Exercise Physiology
- Exercise Testing
- Program Planning
- Program Evaluation
- First Aid/CPR Instruction
- Business Management
- Business Speech
- Personal Computers
- Business Law
- Management
- Industrial Psychology
- Marketing
- Accounting
- Business Statistics
- Medical Records

To further enhance your job prospects, seriously consider a minor in business administration, occupational safety, allied health, or another area related to WHP.

Learn as much as you can about as many things as you can. Read widely from health promotion, fitness, and business publications to keep abreast of today's key issues and trends in WHP (see appendix C on page 165 for a list of publications). To become more liberally educated in the health field, take courses in as many different health-related areas as time allows. A strong knowledge base in the following disciplines will make you much more attractive to employers:

- Aging
- Back health
- Nutrition
- Exercise testing
- Substance abuse
- Managed health care
- Medical self-care
- Demand management
- Adult fitness
- Weight management
- Exercise physiology
- Smoking cessation
- Ergonomics
- Occupational safety

During your senior year, talk to your academic advisor to learn more about certification opportunities, professional conferences, and networking opportunities. Also, be sure to sign up with your university's job placement (career) center. A job placement center can do a lot of work for you in the future, especially if you're applying for many positions. For instance, the center will hold all your letters of recommendation for you and mail them to prospective employees at your request.

CERTIFICATION: A GROWING TREND

As more worksite health and fitness positions require appropriate certification, it's important to select a college or university with a strong academic and skills-development curriculum. Some organizations that offer certification standards for many colleges and universities are listed in appendix C (p. 165).

When inquiring about the quality of specific certification programs, ask your advisor or the certifying organization these questions:

- How desirable are your certifications in the marketplace?
- What distinguishes one certification from others?
- What type of academic background and technical skills should applicants have prior to a certification test?

- Is there an ongoing program in place that promotes continued competence (e.g., continuing education units)?

- Does at least one public member serve on the governing board of the organization?

- Is there a formal disciplinary policy designed to protect the public from unethical or unwarranted certification?

INTERNSHIPS

One of the best ways to increase your marketability is to gain worksite experience before entering the job market. Many businesses, industries, health clubs, and health care organizations offer **internships,** which can provide valuable experience in developing and refining your skills in an actual worksite. One student reflects upon his internship:

This internship has been a wonderful learning experience for me. It showed me that I could interact with a wide array of people and help them meet their special needs. I also benefited from my exposure to the employee health screenings, which I would not have gotten through the university. This experience helped hone my writing skills, made me more self-reliant (due in part to newly developed computing skills), and increased my self-confidence. I have recognized my shortcomings, too—frustration at

setbacks and the need to prepare further in advance. Overall, this internship was a period of tremendous growth, both professionally and personally. A contributing factor to my growth was the amount of hands-on experience we student interns received.

If you're interested in trying an internship, ask your academic advisor about internship opportunities. You can discuss such factors as geographic preferences, types of worksites you prefer, your career plans, writing an application letter, living arrangements, university policies regarding internships, preinternship skill development, and so forth.

APPLYING FOR INTERNSHIPS

Although each internship location has its own admission criteria, many worksites place emphasis on a prospect's

- ability to perform basic health screenings (e.g., body fat, blood pressure, flexibility),

- grade point average of B or better in major field of study,

- evidence of a proven work ethic (e.g., volunteering, summer jobs),

- certification in first aid and CPR,

- good written and verbal communication skills, and

- evidence of a healthy lifestyle and image.

INTERNSHIP OPPORTUNITIES

Don't neglect to . . .

- discuss possible internship sites with your major advisor
- consult one or more of the following internship directories:

AWHP Annual Directory
Association for Worksite Health Promotion
60 Revere Drive, Suite 500
Northbrook, IL 60012
(847) 480-9574

Career Services Bulletin
American College of Sports Medicine
P.O. Box 1440
Indianapolis, IN 46206-1440
(317) 637-9200

Job Opportunities Bulletin
National Wellness Association
1045 Clark Street, Suite 210
Stevens Point, WI 54481
(800) 244-8922

Many worksites provide a standard application form for intern prospects to submit. A sample application may request

- information about your major and minor fields of study,

- your grade point average,

- the type of internship site desired (manufacturing industry, hospital, small business, managed care organization, community health organization, health club, rehabilitation center, etc.),

- your certifications,

- dates of your proposed internship,

- number of hours per week required by the university,

- major and minor courses completed,

- goals you would like to achieve in an internship,

- your greatest strengths and weaknesses, and

- other information that you believe an internship supervisor and staff members should know about you.

Before offering you an internship, a worksite may require a personal interview, but a phone interview may be acceptable for out-of-state candidates.

INTERNSHIP GUIDELINES

Internship experiences vary widely from site to site. For most students, an internship is the only real worksite experience they have before entering the job market. Thus, internships should feature clear policies and procedures. For example, the *Student Worksite Health Promotion Manual* developed by the author includes guidelines defining the relationship between student interns, university supervisors, and worksite supervisors. Here is a condensed version of these guidelines:

1. Most worksites require interns to have personal liability insurance coverage. This coverage is typically available through the university's personnel or human resources department at a very low cost.

2. The operating procedures of each internship are subject to both the worksite's discretion and the university's policies.

3. With rare exceptions, interns must pay their own expenses (housing, transportation, meals, etc.).

4. Interns should experience the responsibilities of a full-time employee. Thus, a variety of activities are encouraged to foster an appreciation of the commitment required for a full-time job.

5. A university supervisor will normally visit the employer at least once to observe and discuss the intern's performance. Telephone conversations may be used in place of on-site visits at distant locations.

6. The internship should last at least 10 weeks, with an average workload of 40 hours per week.

7. A successfully completed internship is worth 12 semester hours of credit.

COMMON REQUIREMENTS FOR INTERNS

Sponsoring worksites and universities generally specify responsibilities for student interns. Some common work requirements for interns include the following:

1. Completing a basic orientation to the organization with a primary focus on

- its organizational (corporate) hierarchy,

- major health promotion programs and services,

- WHP personnel,

- problems, needs, and constraints of the existing health promotion program, and

- duties of an intern.

2. Participate in or observe a variety of ongoing activities, such as staff conferences, workshops, seminars, and health fairs.

3. Complete a Planning and Evaluation Form before starting your major project; review it with the worksite supervisor on a regular basis.

4. If requested, toward the end of your internship, formally present the internship experience to the worksite staff.

To fulfill written requirements for academic credit, the intern is usually responsible for the following:

1. Keeping a daily report of major activities and perceptions.

2. Preparing a weekly one-to-two-page typed paper (based on daily reports) that describes significant events and insights for each week. Give

one copy to the worksite supervisor and mail or fax one to the university supervisor. The worksite supervisor and intern meet weekly to discuss each paper's contents and strategies for overall improvement.

3. Preparing a typed final report that includes both descriptive and analytical material. The first part should include descriptions of

- the organizational structure of the company,
- purposes and goals of the company's health promotion program,
- program components and their functions,
- major sources of funding for the program, and
- project planning and evaluation.

The analytical overview of the internship should include insights on

- being a health promoter in a worksite setting,
- major benefits of the internship,
- suggestions for how the university might improve preinternship training experiences and future internship experiences, and

- how the worksite might improve the internship experience for future interns.

On the final day of your internship, submit two typed, bound copies of the final report—one to the worksite supervisor and one to the university supervisor.

JOB SEEKING

Since competition increases every year, you should position yourself for the job market as early as possible. Register with the on-campus career placement office at least 6 months before you graduate to take advantage of various seminars on interviewing and job seeking. In addition, before graduating, be sure to do the following:

- Ask selective faculty members and your employer (if you are working) to write recommendation letters for you.
- Subscribe to the Sunday edition of a large newspaper from the area in which you hope to work; review the classified jobs section for employment opportunities.

SUPERVISOR RESPONSIBILITIES

Common Responsibilities for Worksite Supervisors

1. Provide the recommended orientation for the intern.
2. Assist in planning intern activities and supervising the intern during the internship.
3. Hold a weekly conference with the intern to discuss the internship experience (overall performance and specific recommendations for improvement).
4. Discuss the intern's performance with the university supervisor at regular intervals.
5. Assist the university supervisor in conducting a midinternship evaluation and final internship evaluation, and recommend a final grade.

Typical Responsibilities for University Supervisors

1. Meet with the prospective intern on several occasions to determine professional interests, skills, and weaknesses; suggest specific preinternship preparatory experiences; investigate worksite options; and coordinate the application process.
2. Clarify assignments and needs with the intern and worksite supervisor.
3. Make one or more visits to the worksite to review weekly progress and conduct midinternship and final internship evaluations.
4. Obtain a letter grade recommendation from the worksite supervisor, grade the intern's final report, and submit a final grade.

- Attend a regional or national convention that includes a job placement center or job fair.

- Join a professional association or job listing vendor to receive listings of new health/fitness positions. Some of the associations in appendix C (p. 165) have job listing services for entry-level and advanced-level job candidates.

PREPARING FOR A JOB INTERVIEW

Review the interview tips and recommendations in the box below. Consider possible questions from the interview and rehearse your answers ahead of time. After practicing on your own, have a friend or classmate play the role of a prospective employer and ask you typical interview questions (along with a few surprises).

KNOW YOUR COMPANY

In the weeks and days before your interview, discover as much as you can about your potential future employer. Try to learn these specifics:

- Size of the company (number of employees and number of sites)

- Potential growth of the company

- Products, programs, and services the company provides

- Organizational structure of company headquarters and division offices or plants

- Management style (authoritative, participative, or a mixture)

- Union status (and relationship between union and management)

- Recent news about the company

- Company's health promotion philosophy

- Health promotion programs and facilities already in place

- Major health problems of an organization's work-force

- Organizational structure of health and fitness and safety personnel; level of integration

- Potential growth of health promotion programs.

Much of this information can be found in the company's annual report. Request a copy from the company or look for one at your local library. Also consult other library materials, such as *Standard & Poor's Directory.*

INTERVIEW LIKE A PROFESSIONAL

- Dress professionally and arrive a few minutes early for the interview.
- Greet the interviewer with a handshake and pleasant smile.
- Maintain good posture and a calm disposition throughout the interview.
- In case your interviewer is not as organized as you are, bring along a clean copy of your resume for the interviewer to have on hand.
- Give the interviewer enough time to ask each question completely. Take time to think about the question before responding.
- Be honest—most interviewers will see through phoniness.
- Avoid overusing technical terms (the interviewer might think you are pretentious).
- Avoid hand motions and other emphatic gestures.
- Send a letter of appreciation to the interviewer within 2 days after the interview.

WHP Resources

WORLDWIDE WEBSITES

Organization	Address
American Cancer Society	www.cancer.org
American Heart Association	www.amhrt.org
American Lung Association	www.lungusa.org
Association for WHP	www.awhp.com
Centers for Disease Control	www.cdc.gov
Federal Government	www.healthfinder.gov
Food & Drug Administration	www.fda.gov
Gatorade Sport Science Institute	www.gssiweb.com
National Health Information Center	http://nhic-nt.health.org
National Institute on Drug Abuse	www.nida.nih.gov
National Library of Medicine (National Institutes of Health)	www.nlm.nih.gov
Occupational Safety and Health Administration	www.osha.gov
Wellness Councils of America	www.welcoa.org
WellTech International	www.welltech.com/ workplacehealth
World Health Organization	www.december.com/ web/text

Topic-Specific

AIDS/HIV	www.caps.uscf.edu/capsweb
Dietary guidelines	odphp.oash.dhhs.gov/pubs/ dietguid/default.htm
Drugs	www.nida.nih.gov
Ergonomics	www.ergoweb.com
Fitness	www.fitnesslink.com
Healthy People 2000	http://158.72.20.10/ pubs/hp2000/

Organization	Address
Mental Health	www.apa.org
Occupational stress	www.workhealth.org/ prevent/prred.htm
Resources	www.siu.edu/departments/bushea
Surgeon General's Report on Physical Activity	www.cdc.gov/nccdphp/ sgr/sgr.htm
Weight Control/Nutrition	www.eatright.org

HIV/AIDS RESOURCES

AIDS Education in the Workplace (video and booklet) $398. Proceeds support HIV-AIDS education.

AIDS Foundation
P.O. Box 6182
San Francisco, CA 94101-6182
(415) 863-AIDS

AIDS, the Family, and the Community (26-minute video, #2346) $149 (or $75 to rent)
AIDS: Our Worst Fears (28-minute video, #1052) $159 (or $75 to rent)

Films for the Humanities & Sciences
P.O. Box 2053
Princeton, NJ 08543-2053
(800) 257-5126

American Red Cross
Contact your local chapter for information about its workplace HIV-AIDS program.

Citizens' Commission on AIDS for New York City and Northern New Jersey
121 Avenue of the Americas, Sixth Floor
New York, NY 10013
(212) 925-5290

National AIDS Hotline
(800) 342-AIDS

National AIDS Information Clearinghouse
P.O. Box 6003
Rockville, MD 20850
(800) 458-5231

The Small Business Response to AIDS Project
NOVA Healthcare Group
7661 Provincial Drive, Suite 209
McLean, VA 22102
(703) 448-0890

Drug Abuse Prevention and Employee Assistance Programs

EAP Digest
Performance Resource Press, Inc.
1863 Technology Drive
Troy, MI 48083-4244
(810) 588-7733

Employee Assistance
Stevens Publishing Co.
P.O. Box 2573
Waco, TX 76702-2523
(817) 776-9000

National Institute on Drug Abuse Hotline
CEOs and managers can call 1-800-843-4971 to find out how to set up a worksite program for drug abuse prevention.

The U.S. Journal of Drug and Alcohol Dependence
U.S. Journal & Health Communications
3201 S.W. 15th Street
Deerfield Beach, FL 33442
(800) 851-9100

Workplace Drug Abuse Policy, Dept. of Health and Human Services (ADM) 89-1610
Office of Workplace Initiatives, NIDA
Room 10A-54
5600 Fishers Lane
Bethesda, MD 20857
(301) 443-6780

Ergonomics
Workplace Ergonomics
P. O. Box 713
Mt. Morris, IL 61054-0713
(815) 734-1159

Nutrition
American Dietetic Association
216 West Jackson Blvd., Suite 800
Chicago, IL 60606-6995
(312) 899-0040

National Heart, Lung, and Blood Institute
Coordinator for Workplace Activities
Office of Prevention, Education and Control
Bldg. 31, Room 4A18
Bethesda, MD 20892
(301) 496-4236

Nutrition News
National Dairy Council
6300 North River Road
Rosemont, IL 60018
(847) 803-2000

Society for Nutrition Education
1736 Franklin Street
Oakland, CA 94612
(415) 444-7133

Worksite Nutrition: A Decision-Maker's Guide
Office of Disease Prevention and Health Promotion (ODPHP)
P.O. Box 1133
Washington, DC 20013-1133
(800) 336-4797

Smoking Control
Action on Smoking and Health
2013 H Street, N.W.
Washington, DC 20006
(202) 659-4310

American Cancer Society
Model Policy for Smoking in the Workplace
Contact your local ACS office.

American Heart Association
Heart at Work: A Wellness Guide
Contact your local AHA office.

American Lung Association
On the Air—A Guide to Creating a Smoke-free Workplace
Contact your local ALA office.

Institute for Occupational Smoking Policy
The Albers School of Business
Seattle University
Seattle, WA 98122
(206) 296-5700

National Interagency Council on Smoking and Health
291 Broadway
New York, NY 10007
(212) 227-4390

U.S. Office on Smoking and Health
Park Bldg., Room 1-10
5600 Fishers Lane
Rockville, MD 20857
(301) 443-5287

Medical Self-Care and Consumerism
 HealthyLife Self-Care Guide
American Institute for Preventive Medicine
30445 Northwestern Highway, Suite 350
Farmington Hills, MI 48334
(810) 539-1800

Healthwise Handbook
Healthwise, Inc.
P.O. Box 1989
Boise, ID 83701
(208) 345-1161

Prepared for Health Care: A Consumer's Guide to Better Medical Decisions
Mosby-Great Performance, Inc.
14964 N.W. Greenbrier Pkwy.
Beaverton, OR 97006
(800) 433-3803

Self-Care Catalog
5850 Shellbound Avenue
Emeryville, CA 94662-0813
(800) 345-3371

Self-Care: Relief for Common Symptoms
Krames Communications, Inc.
1100 Grundy Lane
San Bruno, CA 94066-3030
(800) 333-3032

Take Care of Yourself
The Center for Corporate Health
10467 White Granite Drive, Suite 300
Oakton, VA 22124
(703) 218-8406

Well Advised: Your Guide to Total Health Care
Park Nicollet Medical Foundation
3800 Park Nicollet Blvd.
Minneapolis, MN 55416
(800) 372-7776
        or

Mosby Consumer Health
11830 Westline Industrial Blvd.
St. Louis, MO 63146
(800) 433-3803

WORKSITE HEALTH PROMOTION RESOURCE VENDORS

There are hundreds of vendors that sell or provide commercialized WHP materials. A sample listing of vendors follows:

American Institute for Preventive Medicine
30445 Northwestern Hwy., Suite 350
Farmington Hills, MI 48334
(810) 539-1800

Health Awareness, Inc.
2262 Cumberland
Rochester Hills, MI 48301
(810) 651-3430

Health Edco, Inc.
P. O. Box 21207
Waco, TX 76702-9964
(800) 299-3366, ext. 295

Health Promotion Services, Inc.
6488 Thunderbird Drive
Indian Head Park, IL 60525
(888) 246-8008

HOPE Publications
350 E. Michigan Avenue, Suite 301
Kalamazoo, MI 49007
(616) 343-0770

Krames Communications
110 Grundy Lane, Suite 224
San Bruno, CA 94066-3030
(800) 333-3032

Mosby Consumer Health
11830 Westline Industrial Drive
St. Louis, MO 63146
(800) 433-3803

Occupational Health Strategies, Inc./ Healthy Achievers
22 Hayes Road
Madbury, NH 03820
(603) 743-3838

Parlay International
P.O. Box 8817
Emeryville, CA 94662-0817
(800) 457-2752

Society for Nutrition Education
1736 Franklin Street
Oakland, CA 94612
(415) 444-7133

StayWell Health Management Systems, Inc.
1340 Mendota Heights Road
St. Paul, MN 55120-1128
(612) 454-3577

HEALTH ASSOCIATIONS AND ORGANIZATIONS

There are more than 200 health-related associations and organizations in the U.S. alone, and most offer inexpensive (or free) user-friendly resources for general health information. Look in the local yellow pages or order a printed listing of private and public sources for $17.25 from Resource Information Guide, P.O. Box 990297, Redding, CA 96099.

The National Health Information Center at (800) 336-4797 can also refer you to the appropriate organization to answer questions or discuss your concerns.

For women's illnesses, the **National Women's Health Network** (202) 347-1140 provides information and referrals on 75 topics.

Hot Line Connections. For a list of 100 hot lines on various illnesses, call the **National Health Information Center** at (800) 336-4797. For $1, it will send a roster of toll-free health information numbers.

SUPPORT GROUPS

The American Self-Help Clearinghouse at St. Clares-Riverside Medical Center in Denville, N.J., tracks more than 700 groups and publishes the *Self-Help Sourcebook*, which is available for $10. (201) 625-7101.

The National Self-Help Clearinghouse will send a list of support group information. Send a self-addressed, stamped envelope to 24 West 43rd St., New York, NY 10036. (212) 354-8525.

COMPUTER-SEARCH RESOURCES

There are more than 245 databases of computerized indexes of information on health issues and promotion. Most searches are based on **Medline**, a data-

base of 3,600 medical journals. A *Medline* search costs $48. With a personal computer, modem, and software package ("Grateful Med"), the caller can conduct a search for in-depth articles on any medical subject. For the Grateful Med software, call (800) 638-8480; for a free demo disk and brochure, call (310) 496-6308. For a guide to other databases, the **Directory of Online Healthcare Databases** is available for $38. (503) 471-1627.

Computer bulletin boards scan exchanges between people delving into various medical subjects. For a list of health-oriented computer bulletin boards, send $5 and a self-addressed, stamped envelope to **Black Bag BBS**, 1 Ball Farm Way, Wilmington, DE 19809; with a modem, dial (302) 994-3772.

Data Brokers. These rely heavily on MEDLINE, tend to be consumer oriented, and are staffed by professionals:

- **The Medical Data Exchange** offers a search on its own consumer health database, *MDX Health Digest,* for $25. Call (503) 471-1627
- **The Medical Information Service** of the Palo Alto Medical Foundation (800) 999-1999
- **Planetree Health Resource Center** (415) 923-3680

RESOURCES FOR SMALL BUSINESSES

American Heart Association. More than 3,000 companies have used AHA's "Heart at Work" program. Employers can choose one or more of five modules. The program covers different aspects of cardiovascular health: high blood pressure; smoking cessation; nutrition and weight control; exercise; and warning signals of heart problems and basic emergency treatment. Contact your local AHA.

American Lung Association. ALA's "Freedom From Smoking" educational campaign involves eight smoking cessation clinics, self-help manuals, videos, and promotional materials. Manuals and videos may be purchased separately. ALA's "Team Up for Freedom from Smoking" incorporates policy development, promotional materials, and motivational items to encourage people to stop smoking. Contact your local ALA.

Asthma and Allergy Foundation of America. The foundation's Asthma Care Training program was first offered to employers in 1988. It is designed for 7 to 12-year-old children to reduce the frequency and severity of asthmatic attacks. Through five 1-hour meetings, the program helps children and parents better recognize warning symptoms and modify behavior accordingly. For more information, contact: AAFA, 1125 15th Street, N.W., Suite 502, Washington, DC 20005. (800) 727-8462.

Blue Cross/Blue Shield's (New Hampshire) Healthy Employees Lifestyles Program (HELP). Health promotion programs and services are available to small and large worksites. For more information, contact: Health Promotion Department, Blue Cross and Blue Shield of New Hampshire, Two Pillsbury Street, Concord, NH 03306. (603) 224-9511, ext. 2762.

March of Dimes. The program "Babies & You" is offered at three levels: (1) an informational campaign that provides companies with posters, brochures, and paycheck stuffers; (2) nine seminars on factors that affect pregnancy, such as nutrition, exercise, age, and genetics; and (3) a personnel training program that enables companies to incorporate "Babies & You" into their health promotion programs. For more information, contact: March of Dimes Birth Defects Foundation at (800) 367-6630.

PROGRAM PLANNING GUIDES

Health Insurance: It's Everybody's Business. A Guide for Small Business Owners. A free brochure. Contact Health Insurance Association of America, 1025 Connecticut Avenue, N.W., Washington, DC, 20036-3998. (202) 824-1600.

Wellness at Work: A Practical Guide for Health Promotion in Small Business. Contact: Wellness Councils of America (WELCOA), Community Health Plaza, 7101 Newport Avenue, Suite 311, Omaha, NE, 68152. (402) 572-3590.

Media Report on Small Business. Contact: Washington Business Group on Health, 777 N. Capitol Street, S.E., Washington, DC, 20002. (202) 408-9320.

Presentation Outlines

The following presentation outlines are designed for worksite health personnel to consider when doing "Lunch 'n Learn" seminars, one-on-one counseling sessions, and small group presentations.

Topic: **Exercise**

Title: **Energizing for Life**

Content Outline

A. Establish incentives for exercising, such as:

- Enhance physical appearance
- Socialize with others
- Manage mental stress
- Lower heart disease risk

B. Preview important terms, such as the following, by defining and giving examples of each:

- Aerobic
- Cardiovascular
- Cardiorespiratory
- Physical fitness
- Resting heart rate
- Maximum heart rate
- Target zone
- Activity training pattern
- Training effect

C. Describe how aerobic exercise helps the major organs, muscles, and tissues in the body:

- Arteries remain elastic longer
- More blood pumped by heart
- More oxygen used by lungs
- Resting heart rate usually drops

- Blood sugar (glucose) drops
- "Good" cholesterol (HDL) increases

D. Preview important steps in developing a personal exercise program. Before helping someone start a program, ask him or her to answer the following questions.

1. Have you ever had . . .

A heart attack?	High blood pressure?
A heart problem?	Diabetes?
Angina pectoris (chest pain)?	A thyroid problem?

2. Do you smoke?
3. Were you born with a congenital heart disease or other heart problem?
4. Have you had surgery in the past year?
5. Are you currently taking any medication?
6. Are you more than 30 pounds overweight?
7. If you are female, are you currently pregnant?

If you answered *yes* to any of the questions above, discuss your exercise plans with your doctor before beginning a program.

E. Help individuals choose the most appropriate type of exercise.

If you want to . . .

Lose weight	Consider aerobic exercises such as: walking, running, swimming, aerobics, cycling
Relieve stress	Do any aerobic exercise
Increase your endurance	Gradually increase the duration of aerobic exercise
Increase your flexibility	Swim, dance, and do easy stretches

F. Instruct on how to warm up properly. Remind exercisers not to bounce while stretching.

G. Getting a program under way:

1. Show how to determine MHR (maximum heart rate)—for example, a 40-year-old has a MaxHR of 180 beats per minute. MHR is determined by subtracting your age from 220.

2. From your MHR, determine your safe target zone. For example,

$180 \times 60 = 108$ (minimum desired heart rate)
$180 \times 85 = 153$ (maximum desired heart rate)

Target zone is 108 to 153.

3. Describe the training effect of exercising in the target zone for at least 15 to 20 continuous minutes, several times per week:

- Heart muscle becomes stronger.
- Blood vessels maintain elasticity.
- Lungs use oxygen more efficiently.

H. Describe how the preceding components can be integrated into a personal exercise program.

I. Explain a postactivity pulse check (to check for overexertion).

Teaching Aids

Note that **B** below corresponds with **B** in the previous section, and so on.

B. Use transparencies, slides, posters, and other materials to illustrate basic anatomy (heart, lungs, blood vessels). Use an animal heart to illustrate the cardiovascular system and coronary arteries.

C. Use a rubber band to show how a blood vessel stretches during exercise.

D. Show questions on a transparency, slide, or handout.

F. Use a transparency or chart to illustrate key muscle groups.

G. Use a transparency or poster to illustrate how to determine MHR and target zone. Draw or illustrate effects using visual aids such as making a squeezed fist (heart pumping more blood with

fewer strokes), balloon (lung capacity), and rubber band (blood vessel elasticity).

H. Illustrate the "activity training pattern" on a transparency and describe how MHR, target zone, and pulse taking relate to the pattern.

Group Activities

A. Ask group members to discuss why they do or do not exercise regularly.

D. Consider each question and explain its intent. For example, chest pains may not always indicate a heart attack. Ask group members to identify what activities cause them chest pain.

E. Have group members develop personal goals. The instructor can suggest the most appropriate exercise.

F. Instructor demonstrates proper warm-up technique for each muscle group and the importance of gradual, gentle stretching without pain.

G. Have each person calculate his or her minimum and maximum heart rate.

H. Instructor leads group in a 10- to 15-minute walk; instruct individuals when to take pulses.

I. Have individuals wait 30 minutes after finishing the walk and take pulse ("recovery pulse"); if pulse is 10 or more beats above resting pulse, the length or pace of the walk was probably too strenuous for these individuals. Instructor should advise them to work up gradually to walking 20 to 30 minutes nonstop at a moderate pace at least 5 days a week.

Topic: **Resistance Training**
Title: **Muscling In**
Content Outline

A. Establish incentives for improving muscular strength and endurance through resistance training:

1. Improve posture
2. Increase lean body mass
3. Increase muscular strength and endurance

4. Improve agility

5. Increase Basal Metabolic Rate (BMR): helps burn more calories

B. Preview important terms by defining and giving examples of the following:

- Strength
- Muscular endurance
- Power
- Hypertrophy
- Atrophy
- Concentric
- Eccentric
- Isometric exercise
- Isotonic exercise
- Isokinetic exercise
- Circuit training
- Plyometric training

C. Describe the anatomy and physiology of skeletal muscles

1. Four characteristics of skeletal muscles:

   Elasticity   Excitability

   Extensibility   Contractility

2. Large muscles produce gross motor movements at large joints, such as the knee.

3. Smaller muscles produce fine motor movements, such as those in the fingers.

D. Methods of improving muscular strength and endurance

1. Muscular strength gains are achieved using heavier weights with a lower number of repetitions (3 sets of 6 to 10 reps).

2. Muscular endurance gains are achieved using lighter weights with a greater number of repetitions (3 sets of 10 to 12 reps).

3. Isometric exercise . . .

   - involves a contraction of the muscle in which the length of the muscle remains constant.

   - involves contraction against some immovable resistance.

   - tends to increase blood pressure, which can result in a fatal cardiovascular attack in susceptible individuals.

4. Isotonic exercise . . .

   - involves a contraction in which force is produced as the muscle changes in length.

   - often involves using free weights, dumbbells, and barbells.

   - involves *concentric* contraction, which is shortening of the muscle.

   - involves *eccentric* contraction is the lengthening of the muscle.

5. Isokinetic exercise . . .

   - involves a contraction in which the length of the muscle is changing while maximal resistance is provided throughout the entire contraction.

   - often involves using Cybex, Lido, and KinCom exercise machines.

   - is often done during rehabilitation.

E. Techniques of Muscular Training

1. Circuit training . . .

   - is a series of exercise stations combining resistance training, flexibility, and brief aerobic exercises.

   - usually consists of 8 to 12 stations with about 30 seconds spent at each and the entire circuit repeated 3 times.

2. In plyometric training . . .

   - a brief eccentric stretch of a muscle is immediately followed by a concentric contraction of the same muscle.

   - the quick stretch of a muscle produces a reflex contraction of the muscle in response to the stretch.

F. Teaching Aids

1. Transparencies illustrating various resistance training equipment and methods

2. Transparency illustrating major muscles of the body

3. Transparency illustrating the different muscle contractions

4. Use a dumbbell to demonstrate exercises to target all major muscle groups:

   - Chest press
   - Bent-over row (back)
   - Biceps curl
   - Triceps extension

- Shoulder press
- Squats/lunges (thighs/buttocks)
- Toe raises (calves)
- Crunches (abdominals)

5. Use a box to demonstrate plyometric training.

6. Use a stopwatch, jump rope, and dumbbells to demonstrate circuit training.

G. Miscellaneous

1. Breathe properly during exercise.

2. You don't need to join a health club—push-ups and dips are great upper body exercises. You can improvise by using "homemade" equipment, such as soup cans instead of dumbbells.

Topic: Stress Management

Title: Taking Charge of Your Life!

Content Outline

A. Definition of *stress* is "external force causing internal changes." External forces are called *stressors.*

B. Identify common stressors, such as:

- Children
- Personal expectations
- Finances
- Others (list)
- Job

C. Help group members acknowledge mental or physical signals during stress, such as:

- Increased heart rate
- Headache
- Increased breathing
- Nervousness
- Muscle tension
- Others (list)

D. Help group members learn stress-management techniques such as:

- Relaxation response
- Yoga
- Progressive relaxation
- Controlled breathing

Teaching Aids

A. Show a short video illustrating common types of stress.

Group Activities

A. Preview video before you show it; review the video's major highlights after showing it.

B. Ask each person to write his or her most common stress-producing events (stressors) on paper and voluntarily share with others.

C. Have members voluntarily describe major stress signals.

Techniques and Procedures

Relaxation Response

1. Sit or lie in a comfortable position in a quiet environment with eyes closed.

2. Beginning with the feet, relax each muscle group in the following order: calf-thigh-waist; stomach-arms-chest; neck-face-forehead. Say to yourself, "My muscles are very relaxed."

3. Breathe in through the nose, hold, and exhale through your mouth. As you inhale, gently push your stomach out 2 to 4 inches (no chest movement); as you exhale, allow your stomach to flatten.

4. Continue for several minutes.

Progressive Relaxation

1. Lie flat on a soft surface or floor with your eyes closed and knees bent.

2. Beginning with your right foot, press foot firmly to the floor for 5 seconds—relax for 5 seconds; repeat with left foot.

3 Straighten legs out and press back of lower right leg firmly to the floor for 5 seconds—relax for 5 seconds; repeat with left leg.

4. Press each of the following areas firmly to the floor for 5 seconds—relax for 5 seconds (one at a time):

- back of thigh and buttocks
- lower back—shoulder blades
- arms
- back of head

5. Breathe normally as you press and relax.

Yoga (a series of rhythmic movements held for a few seconds)

1. Stand relaxed, arms hanging at sides and feet about one foot apart.

2. Tilt head back and hold for 5 seconds.

3. Roll head forward and hold for 5 seconds.

4. Curl chest and stomach forward as you bend at the waist; arms dangling for 5 seconds.

5. Inhale slowly through mouth as you straighten up. Raise arms overhead; drop arms slowly to sides as you exhale slowly through mouth.

Controlled Breathing

1. Lie down with your back flat on the floor; place a book or large magazine on your stomach.

2. Bend your knees and close your eyes.

3. Push your stomach up 2 to 3 inches and hold for 5 seconds, then exhale. Repeat several times. Each time you exhale, say "I am relaxed." Avoid lifting your chest.

The diaphragm is the major breathing muscle and is located between your chest and belly button.

Topic: **Weight Management**
Title: **Controlling Weight for Life**

Content Outline

A. Establish incentives for controlling body weight

B. Outline the components of the body

- height
- lean muscle
- body fat percentage
- body type
  endomorph (muscular)
  ectomorph (thin)
  mesomorph (average)

C. Preview important terms by defining and giving examples of the following terms:

- self-esteem
- set point
- fat cells (adipocytes)
- fad diet
- yo-yo dieting
- weight control
- nutrition
- calorie
- basal metabolic rate
- obesity
- behavior modification
- body mass index
- energy
- metabolism
- overweight
- balanced diet

D. Physical Assessments:

1. Explain how some Recommended Body Weight tables may be invalid due to skewed representation (i.e., smokers typically weigh less and die prematurely resulting in a higher percentage of heavier nonsmokers whose weights inflate the desirable weight levels).

2. Explain the difference between body weight and body fat percentage and that many physically fit persons can be overweight due to having a lot of muscle (mostly water), but not overfat.

E. How to modify diet and exercise for permanent weight control.

Teaching Aids

B. Use a transparency to illustrate various people of different sizes and shapes

C. Posters, calculators

D. Recommended body weight chart, weight scales, skinfold calipers, personal data sheet to record body weight and body fat percentage

E. Illustrate how to establish a reasonable eating plan combined with exercise; food models (plastic or rubber) can be shown with an overview of the nutritional value of the various foods. Supply a daily eating and exercise diary.

Group Activities

D. Voluntary: interested persons may have their body weight and body fat percentage calculated for them.

E. Have participants develop personal goals to share with appropriate health professionals.

Topic: **Medical Self-Care**
Title: **Taking Care of Yourself!**

Content Outline

A. Establish incentives (reasons) for using self-care such as:

- treating a minor condition before it can worsen

- saving time by not waiting in line at a doctor's office or emergency room

- spending less money out-of-pocket on health care

- fewer health care dollars spent by your employer

- others (list): _____

_____

_____

B. Explain various health care options for treating minor ailments

- personal physician

- worksite nurse/doctor

- self-care

Teaching Aids

A. Use handouts, transparencies, slides, posters and other resources to illustrate the basic principles of self-care. Distribute a personal copy of a self-care book to all participants.

Group Activities

A. Ask group members to explain why they do or do not use the worksite medical department/doctor for simple health problems, i.e., sore throat, upset stomach, etc. . . .

B. Ask participants to select a common health problem in the book. Explain the proper treatment, then ask one participant to select another problem for which group members can identify the appropriate self-care teatment in the book. Consider a team competition (department vs. department) and reward the winners.

Topic: Nutrition

Title: Eating for Energy!

Content Outline

A. Establish reasons for eating well-balanced meals:

- energy
- reduce health risks
- good health

B. Define and give examples of key terms:

- protein
- carbohydrates
- fat
- saturated
- unsaturated
- polyunsaturated
- vitamins
- minerals
- trace elements

C. Dietary Assessment:

Compare examples of actual caloric intake vs. desirable calorie intake

D. Describe various ways to prepare a healthy eating plan. For the average person:

- reduce total and saturated fat intake

- reduce sugar intake

- increase fiber intake

E. Reading a nutrition label; explain what is required on a label

Teaching Aids

B. Show USDA food pyramid and describe what types of foods fit in each category. Provide examples with plastic/rubber models of various foods.

D. In addition to models of food, posters, etc., distribute real food samples (fruit, bagels, etc.).

E. Distribute copies of an actual label.

Group Activities

B. Have participants complete a dietary intake record of the past 2 to 3 days.

C. Do a computerized nutritional analysis of each record to identify deficiencies and excesses.

D. Ask participants to identify various foods that can be used in a healthy eating plan.

E. Distribute a second label and ask participants to identify key information of greatest value to consumers.

Topic: Back Health

Title: Back to Good Health!

Content Outline

A. Highlight the frequency of low back problems and why the lower back is so vulnerable to injury.

B. Approximately 90 percent of all back pain/ injury episodes improve with minimal or no medical intervention. However, to minimize the risk of future injury, it is important to strengthen the abdominal and back muscles and avoid dangerous habits. Numerous factors increase low back injury risk, e.g., frequent lifting of heavy objects, poor biomechanics, poor work station ergonomics, etc.

C. Explain proper lifting technique.

Teaching Aids

A. Use transparencies, slides, and posters to illustrate the basic anatomy of the spinal column.

C. Use empty boxes.

Group Activities

B. Organize and conduct a sit-and-reach test to assess back flexibility.

C. Organize and conduct a stretching session to focus on appropriate ways to stretch. Demonstrate the correct lifting technique and have participants practice.

Professional Preparation Resources

Professional Associations

Association for Worksite Health Promotion
  (AWHP)
60 Revere Drive, Suite 500
Northbrook, IL 60062
(847) 480-9574; www.awhp.com

American College of Sports Medicine
P.O. Box 1440
Indianapolis, IN 46206-1440
(317) 637-9200; www.acsm.com

National Wellness Association
1300 College Court
P. O. Box 827
Stevens Point, WI 54481
(715) 342-2979; www.wellnessnwi.org

Wellness Councils of America (WELCOA)
7101 Newport Avenue, Suite 311
Omaha, NE 68152
(402) 572-3590; FAX: (402) 572-3594
www.welcoa.org

Organizations Sponsoring Exercise-Specific Certification Programs

Certifying Organization	Types of Certifications
Aerobic Fitness Association of America 15250 Ventura Blvd., Suite 802 Sherman Oaks, CA 91403 (800) 445-5950	Aerobics instruction Step instruction Weight room instruction Personal training Emergency response
American College of Sports Medicine P.O. Box 1440 Indianapolis, IN 46206-1440 (317) 637-9200	Program director Exercise specialist Exercise test technologist Health/fitness director Health/fitness instructor Exercise leader
American Council on Exercise 5820 Oberlin Drive, Suite 102 San Diego, CA 92121-3787 (800) 825-3636	Aerobics instructor Personal trainer Lifestyle/weight management
Association of Worksite Health Promotion 60 Revere Drive, Suite 500 Northbrook, IL 60012 (847) 480-9574	Contact for details

(continued)

Certifying Organization	Types of Certifications
Cooper Institute for Aerobics Research 12330 Preston Road Dallas, TX 75230 (800) 635-7050, ext. 830	Contact for details
Desert Southwest Fitness, Inc. 3202 E. Via Celeste Tucson, AZ 85718 (800) 873-6759	Contact for details
IDEA, The Int'l Association of Fitness 6190 Cornerstone Court, Suite 204 San Diego, CA 92121 (619) 535-8979	Fitness instructors Fitness directors Personal trainers
National Federation of Professional Trainers P.O. Box 4579 Lafayette, IN 47903 (317) 447-3287	Personal training
National Strength & Conditioning Association P.O. Box 38909 Colorado Springs, CO 80937 (402) 476-6669	Strength and conditioning Personal training
The Universal Fitness Institute 930 27th Avenue, S.W. P.O. Box 1270 Cedar Rapids, IA 52406	Contact for details
YMCA of the USA 101 N. Wacker Drive Chicago, IL 60606 (800) 872-9622	Fitness leader Fitness instructor Fitness specialist Strength-training instructor Strength-training director Youth fitness instructor Healthy back instructor Fitness walking instructor Weight-management consultant Prenatal and postpartum exercise instructor

Additional Certification

American Association of Lifestyle Counselors
c/o The LEARN Institute
P.O. Box 35328, Department 50
Dallas, TX 75235-0328
(800) 736-7323
	Certified Lifestyle Counselor in Weight
	   Management
	Certified Lifestyle Counselor in Stress
	   Management

Trade and Professional Publications

ACSM's Health & Fitness Journal
Williams & Wilkins
P.O. Box 23291
Baltimore, MD 21298-9325
(800) 486-5643

AWHP's Worksite Health
Association for Worksite Health Promotion
60 Revere Drive, Suite 500
Northbrook, IL 60062

American Journal of Health Promotion
1812 S. Rochester Road, Suite 200
Rochester Hills, MI 48307-3532

Business & Health
Medical Economics Publishing
5 Paragon Drive
Montvale, NJ 07645

BusinessWeek
McGraw-Hill, Inc.
1221 Avenue of the Americas
New York, NY 10020

Club Industry
Cardinal Business Media, Inc.
1300 Virginia Drive, Suite 400
Fort Washington, PA 19034

Employee Benefits Plan Review
Charles D. Spencer & Associates, Inc.
250 S. Wacker Drive
Chicago, IL 60606-5834

Fitness Management
Leisure Publications, Inc.
3923 West 6th Street
Los Angeles, CA 90020

Fortune
Time, Inc.
Time & Life Bldg.
Rockefeller Center
New York, NY 10020-1393

The Physician and Sports Medicine
P.O. Box 462
Hightstown, NJ 08520-9205

Journal of Occupational Health Nursing
American Occupational Health Nursing
  Association
Charles B. Slack, Inc.
6900 Grove Road
Thorofare, NJ 08086

Journal of Occupational Medicine
American Occupational Medicine Association
2340 S. Arlington Heights Road
Arlington Heights, IL 60005

Occupational Health & Safety
Workplace Ergonomics
3700 I-35
Waco, TX 76706

Association for Worksite Health Promotion (AWHP) Competencies

I. Business Management

A. Technological Applications

1. Identify organization and management data needs common to a worksite health promotion program;

2. Select appropriate computer software and other technologies for a worksite health promotion program; and

3. Integrate technological applications into the program design and worksite environment.

B. Facility and Equipment

4. Develop an effective system for inventory control in a health promotion program;

5. Develop an equipment and facility maintenance schedule for a health promotion program;

6. Identify environmental, structural, and legal design issues that facilitate optimum delivery of health promotion services; and

7. Identify appropriate equipment and space needs.

C. Financial Management

8. Use a budgeting process to develop operating and capital budgets for a health promotion program;

9. Present and defend a budget;

10. Interpret financial statements; and

11. Manage a budget.

D. Organizational Policies and Procedures

12. Determine administrative and program policies and procedures in the worksite environment;

13. Integrate a health promotion program's policies and procedures with those of the company;

14. Update policies and procedures based on current standards; and

15. Describe how to adhere to organizational and professional standards concerning confidentiality of information.

E. Communication

16. Describe the program in a written form suitable for publication in a newsletter, trade journal or peer-reviewed publication;

17. Write appropriate management communications (memos and reports) with acceptable business writing form;

18. Describe and demonstrate the oral presentation skills necessary to deliver an effective presentation;

19. Describe different communication styles that can be used with various audiences (such as management, professionals, employees, or dependents);

20. Develop written and oral proposals for a budget, program, policy statement, business plan, and marketing plan;

21. Write appropriate marketing communication pieces for a health promotion program (press releases, brochures, newsletters, flyers, and bulletin board announcements);

22. Use various methods to facilitate effective meetings (rules of order, facilitating skills, small-group dynamics, agendas, and minutes);

23. Develop, review and analyze an overall communication strategy; and

24. Demonstrate effective interpersonal communication skills.

F. Quality Management and Assurance

25. Develop a strategy that will define for the health promotion program a quality management and assurance process that is consistent with the worksite environment;

26. Define the health promotion employee's role in a quality assurance process;

27. Identify recognized and accepted standards of programming quality;

28. Identify potential liability areas and develop a system for legal and risk management; and

29. Identify and influence the organization's stance on health and safety issues.

G. Marketing

30. Use marketing analysis to implement appropriate health promotion program offerings;

31. Describe an appropriate marketing strategy for the target population; and

32. Describe how to position the health promotion program in its competitive environment.

H. Business Planning

33. Define the mission, goals, and objectives of a health promotion program;

34. Develop a work plan, including action steps and policies to carry out the goals and objectives;

35. Develop health promotion program strategies that are acceptable to the cooperating population;

36. Establish interdepartmental collaboration;

37. Influence the design of a benefit package to support health promotion;

38. Develop a strategic planning process and direct the development of a departmental strategic plan;

39. Develop a strategic planning process and influence positioning of a company through health promotion strategic planning;

40. Establish oneself as the corporate health promotion expert and advocate;

41. Propose new concepts, directions, and opportunities for health promotion; and

42. Describe how business planning is used for evaluating and refining the health promotion program.

II. Program Management

A. Needs Analysis

43. Conduct an audit of the organization's priorities and external and internal resources;

44. Formulate a needs-assessment process;

45. Define a target population;

46. Formulate or identify a cost-effective and appropriate needs-assessment methodology;

47. Collect and analyze organizational data related to the development of the health promotion program;

48. Analyze and synthesize the results of the needs assessment; and

49. Summarize and document the results of the assessment.

B. Program Design

50. Define the program's mission, goals, and objectives utilizing needs-assessment data;

51. Define and prioritize the appropriate mix of services and activities to meet the program's goals and objectives based on the population needs;

52. Identify and interpret the results of important studies and apply those results to program design;

53. Identify relevant model programs and apply the knowledge obtained to program design;

54. Plan an organizational culture, structure, and environment;

55. Develop a plan that effectively accounts for action steps, resource allocation, assignment of personnel, and time frames for accomplishing program objectives;

56. Develop a marketing strategy;

57. Design incentive and motivational reinforcements for the program; and

58. Select the appropriate evaluation design that is consistent with the program's goals, objectives and resources.

C. Program Implementation

59. Implement and follow operational and administrative policies and procedures;

60. Market program services and activities;

61. Deliver program services and activities to assure accessibility and maximum utilization; and

62. Apply process-evaluation procedures and modify the program appropriately.

D. Program Evaluation

63. Apply the appropriate designs for impact and outcome evaluation;

64. Utilize the appropriate methods of data collection and analysis;

65. Interpret the data, draw conclusions, and make recommendations; and

66. Disseminate the results of an evaluation to the appropriate individuals within the organization.

III. Human Resource Management

A. Staffing the Health Promotion Program

67. Determine staffing needs based on a health promotion program plan;

68. Conduct a job analysis;

69. Write a job description;

70. Develop performance standards;

71. Evaluate candidates for a job;

72. Review applications and resumes;

73. Conduct a job interview;

74. Evaluate references;

75. Obtain the approval to hire;

76. Orient new health promotion employees to the job, program, and worksite culture; and

77. Manage staffing changes using proper legal procedures and policies of the organization.

B. Train and Develop Personnel

    78. Determine and evaluate staff training and development needs;

    79. Provide or support training and development opportunities for the staff;

    80. Promote personal and career development; and

    81. Delegate appropriate responsibilities and authority to the staff.

C. Manage Human Resources

    82. Establish goals, objectives, and a work plan with each employee on at least an annual basis;

    83. Provide ongoing feedback to employees and conduct regular performance appraisals;

    84. Prepare staff schedules and assign responsibilities;

    85. Anticipate and resolve conflicts;

    86. Motivate personnel to enhance productivity;

    87. Maintain open communication channels between and among management and employees;

    88. Utilize appropriate leadership styles for specific situations;

    89. Determine the criteria for selection of consultants and vendors;

    90. Identify the need for consultant and vendor services;

    91. Negotiate consultant and vendor services contracts;

    92. Identify and comply with company policies and legal procedures relating to consultants and vendors; and

    93. Evaluate the performance of consultants and vendors.

D. Personal Management

    94. Develop a personal career plan to promote self-development;

    95. Model healthy behaviors; and

    96. Demonstrate service to the profession and the community.

REFERENCES AND SUGGESTED READINGS

CHAPTER 1

Aguiree-Molina, M. and Molina, C. (1990). Ethnic/racial populations and worksite health promotion. *Occupational Medicine: State of the Art Reviews: Worksite Health Promotion*, 5, 789-806.

Anderson, D. and Jose, W. (1987). Employer lifestyle and the bottom line. *Fitness in Business*, 2, 86-91.

Bertera, R. (1991). The effect of behavioral risks on absenteeism and health care costs in the workplace. *Journal of Occupational Medicine*, 33, 1119-1124.

Bialkowski, C. (1991). The future of corporate fitness. *Club Industry, 7,* 5, 33-38.

Chenoweth, D. (1993). *Health care cost management: Strategies for employers.* Dubuque, IA: Brown and Benchmark Publishers.

Chenoweth, D. (1991). *Planning health promotion at the worksite.* 2nd edition. Dubuque, IA: Brown and Benchmark Publishers.

Davis, H. (1988). *Fourteen steps in managing an aging work force.* Lexington, MA: Lexington Books.

Kaman, R. (Editor) (1995). *Worksite health promotion economics: Consensus and analysis.* Champaign, IL: Human Kinetics.

Layden, E. (1995). Get off your rocker. *Fitness Management, 11,* 5, 30.

Opatz, J., Chenoweth, D., and Kaman, R. Economic impact of worksite health promotion. (1991). *First Annual Proceedings of the 1990 Association for Fitness in Business Economic Impact Conference*, 1-10.

Opatz, J. (Editor) (1994). *Economic impact of worksite health promotion.* Champaign, IL: Human Kinetics.

Seidler, S., Young, S., and Beckham, M. (1993). *The worksite health promotion sourcebook.* Washington, D.C.: National Resource Center on Worksite Health Promotion.

Taylor, S. (1992). The changing face of aging. *Journal of Health Care Benefits, 1,* 51-54.

Tenser, J. (1992, Mid-March). Long Term Care Insurance: The Rx for a Graying America. *Business and Health*, 53-58.

Tully, S. (1995, June 12). America's healthiest companies. *Fortune*, pp. 98-106.

U.S. Department of Health and Human Services, Public Health Service. (1991). *Healthy People 2000: National Health Promotion and Disease Prevention Objectives.* Washington, D.C.: U.S. Government Printing Office.

U.S. Deptartment of Labor, Bureau of Labor Statistics (1988). *Projection 2000.* Washington, D.C.: U.S. Government Printing Office.

Woodall, G., Higgins, C., Dunn, J., and Nicholson, T. (1987). Characteristics of the frequent visitor to the industrial medical department and implications for health promotion. *Journal of Occupational Medicine*, 29, 660-664.

Yen, L., Edington, D., and Wittig, P. (1991). Association between health risk appraisal scores and employee medical claims costs in a manufacturing company. *American Journal of Health Promotion*, 6, 1, 46-54.

CHAPTER 2

Bialkowski, C. (1991). The future of corporate fitness. *Club Industry, 7,* 5, 33-38.

Chenoweth, D. (1991). Planning health promotion at the worksite. Madison, WI: Brown and Benchmark Publishers.

Fitzler, S. and Berger, R. (1983). Chelsea back program: one year later. *Occupational Health and Safety, 52,* 7, 52-54.

Main, J. (1986, August 18). Under the spell of the quality gurus. *Fortune,* pp. 30-34.

Ouchi, W. (1981). *Theory Z.* Reading, MA: Addison Wesley Publishing.

The 1990 national executive poll on health care costs and benefits. *Business and Health, 8,* 4, 25-38.

Polakoff, P. (1983). Unions can help trim health costs. *Occupational Health and Safety, 52,* 8, 33-37.

Ross, I. (1986, September 25). Corporations take aim at illiteracy. *Fortune,* p. 49.

Senn, K. et al. Health programs should become family affairs. *Occupational Health and Safety, 52,* 6, 37.

Storlie, J., Baun, W., and Horton, W. (1992). *Guidelines for employee health promotion programs.* Champaign, IL: Human Kinetics Publishers.

Suchman, E. (1967). *Evaluative research.* New York: Russell Sage Foundation.

U.S. Department of Health and Human Services, Public Health Service. (1983). *Worksite health promotion: Some questions and answers to help you get started.* Washington, D.C., pp. 11-13.

CHAPTER 3

Cascio, W. (1987). *Costing human resources: The financial impact of behavior in organizations,* 2nd Edition. Boston, MA: PWS-Kent Publishing.

Gerson, R. (1989). *Marketing health/fitness services.* Champaign, IL: Human Kinetics.

Kaman, R. (1995). *Worksite health promotion economics: Consensus and analysis.* Champaign, IL: Human Kinetics.

Sattler, T. and Mullen, J. (1997). Reducing health care costs. *Fitness Management,* May, 20-21.

Van Camp, S.P. (1995). ACSM offers more than exercise lite. *Fitness Management, 11,* 18.

Yen, L., Edington, D., and Wittig, P. (1991). Association between health risk appraisal scores and employee medical claims costs in a manufacturing company. *American Journal of Health Promotion, 6,* 1, 46-54.

CHAPTER 4

Aguiree-Molina, M. and Molina, C. (1990). Ethnic/racial populations and worksite health promotion. *Occupational Medicine: State of the Art Reviews: Worksite Health Promotion, 5,* 4, 789-806.

Anderson, D. and Jose, W. (1987) Employee lifestyle and the bottom line. *Fitness in Business, 2,* 3, 86-91.

Bernacki, E. and Baun, W. (1984). The relationship of job performance to exercise adherence in a corporate fitness program. *Journal of Occupational Medicine, 26,* 7, 529-531.

Bialkowski, C. (1991). The future of corporate fitness. *Club Industry, 7,* 1991, 94.

Cascio, W. (1987). *Costing human resources: The financial impact of behavior in organizations,* 2nd Edition. Boston, MA: PWS-Kent Publishing.

Chenoweth, D. (1993). *Health care cost management: Strategies for employers,* 2nd Edition. Dubuque, IA: Brown and Benchmark.

Cottrell, R. and Donatelle, R. (1988). Using voluntary agencies, university personnel and company volunteers to implement health promotion programs for small businesses. *Fitness in Business, 3,* 216-219.

Davis, H. (1988). *Fourteen steps in managing an aging work force.* Lexington, MA: Lexington Books.

Findlay, S. (1991, June 13). Cozy pact cuts firms' costs. *USA TODAY,* p. B8.

Gerson, R. (1989). *Marketing health/fitness services.* Champaign, IL: Human Kinetics.

Gibbs, J., Mulvaney D., Henes, C., and Reed, R. (1985). Worksite health promotion: Five-year trend in employee health care costs. *Journal of Occupational Medicine, 27,* 826-830.

Hansen, L. (1991, February). Healthy bonuses that pay off. Reprint from *Business New Hampshire Magazine.*

Horowitz, S. (1987). Effects of a worksite program on absenteeism and health care costs in a small federal agency. *Fitness in Business, 2,* 167-172.

Leavenworth, G. (1994). Four cost-cutting strategies. *Business and Health, 12,* 1, 26-34.

Madlin, N. (1991). Wellness incentives: How well do they work? *Business and Health, 9,* 4, 70-74.

Marion Merrell Dow, Inc. (1995). *The future of corporate health benefits; a national report.* Kansas City, MO.

Medrea, J. (1995). How Champion merged health and family services into its business plan. *AWHP's Worksite Health, 1,* 32-35.

National Resource Center on Worksite Health Promotion. (1991). *Healthy People at Work: Strategies for Employers.* Washington, D.C.

New Mexico Health Systems Agency, Health and Industry Project. (1981). *Employee Health and Fitness Programs: A Guide for New Mexico Employers.* Albuquerque, NM.

Opatz, J., Chenoweth, D. and Kaman, R. Economic Impact of Worksite Health Promotion. (1990). *Proceedings of the first annual association for fitness in business economic impact conference,* Fort Worth, TX.

Repackaging of seminars boosts attendance five-fold at Conoco. (1989). *Club Industry, 5,* 10, 15.

Rudnicki, J. and Wankel, L. (1988). Employee fitness program effects upon long-term fitness involvement. *Fitness in Business, 3,* 123-132.

Smith, R. (1990). Work-place stretching programs reduce costly accidents, injuries. *Occupational Health and Safety, 59,* 3, 24-25.

Taylor, S. (1992). The changing face of aging. *Journal of Health Care Benefits, 1,* 2, 51-54.

U. S. Department of Health and Human Services, Public Health Service. (1991). *Healthy people 2000: National health promotion and disease prevention objectives.* Washington, D.C.: U.S. Government Printing Office.

Woodall, G. et al. (1987). Characteristics of the frequent visitor to the industrial medical department and implications for health promotion. *Journal of Occupational Medicine, 29*, 660-664.

Yen, L., Edington, D., and Wittig, P. (1991) Association between health risk appraisal scores and employee medical claims costs in a manufacturing company. *American Journal of Health Promotion, 6,* 1, 46-54.

CHAPTER 5

Bartz, A. (1976). *Basic statistical concepts in education and the behavioral sciences.* Minneapolis, MN: Burgess Publishing Company.

Campbell, D. and Stanley, J. (1963). *Experimental and quasi-experimental designs for research.* Chicago, IL: Rand McNally College Publishing Company.

Chenoweth, D. (1983). Fitness program evaluation: results with muscle. *Occupational Health and Safety, 52*, 6, 14-17 and 40-42.

Chenoweth, D. (1984). Shaping up health promotion for introduction into a workplace. *Occupational Health and Safety, 53,* 5, 49-54.

Kaman, R. (1995). *Worksite health promotion economics: Consensus and analysis.* Champaign, IL: Human Kinetics.

Kerlinger, F. (1973). *Foundations of behavioral research.* New York: Holt, Rinehart and Winston.

Opatz, J. (Ed., 1994). *Economic impact of worksite health promotion.* Champaign, IL: Human Kinetics.

Suchman, E. (1967). *Evaluative Research.* New York: Russell Sage Foundation.

U.S. Department of Health and Human Services, Public Health Service. (1983). *Worksite health promotion: Some questions and answers to help you get started.* Washington, D.C., 11-13.

Van Dalen, D. (1979). *Understanding educational research: An introduction.* New York: McGraw-Hill Book Company.

Windsor, R. et al. (1984). *Evaluation of health promotion and education programs.* Palo Alto, CA: Mayfield Publishing Company.

CHAPTER 6

A cure for stress? (1987, October 12). *BusinessWeek*, pp. 64-65.

Ameritech searches for Holy Grail' to manage STD, LTD, and workers' compensation. (1997, March). *Employee Benefits Plan Review*, pp. 23-24.

Barnett, A. (1995). Is knowledge really power for patients? *Business and Health, 13*, 5, 29-36.

Biering-Sorenson, F. (1984). Physical measurements as risk indicators for low-back trouble over a one-year period. *Spine, 9*, 106-119.

Bowne, D., Russell, M., Morgan, J., Opterberg, S. and Clark, A. (1984). Reduced disability in an industrial fitness program. *Journal of Occupational Medicine, 26*, 809-816.

Brink, S. (1996, February 12). Beating the odds. *U.S. News and World Report*, pp. 60-68.

Brown, H. (1988). Improving maternal health from the board room. *Business and Health, 6,* 1, 10-12.

Cady, L. (1985). Programs for increasing health and physical fitness of firefighters. *Journal of Occupational Medicine, 27*, 110-114.

Cady, L., Bischoff, D., O'Connell, E. et al. (1979). Strength and fitness and subsequent back injuries in firefighters. *Journal of Occupational Medicine, 21*, 269-272.

Chaffin, D., Herrin, G., and Keyserling, W. (1978). Preemployment strength testing—an updated position. *Journal of Occupational Medicine. 20*, 403-408.

Chenoweth, D. (1993). *Health care cost management: Strategies for employers*, 2nd Edition. Brown and Benchmark Publishing.

Chenoweth, D. (1990). Truckers challenged to use clout to effect health promotion changes. *Occupational Health and Safety, 59*, 46.

Data Watch: Maternity and childbirth costs. (1990) *Business and Health, 8*, 5, 8-9.

Fefer, M. (1992, June 27). What to do about workers' comp. *Fortune*, p. 81.

Fisher, K., Glasgow, R., and Terborg, J. (1990). Worksite smoking cessation: a meta-analysis of long-term quit rates from controlled studies. *Journal of Occupational Medicine, 32*, 429-439.

Fitzler, S. and Berger, R. (1983). Chelsea back program: One year later. *Occupational Health and Safety, 52*, 7, 52-54.

Gates, S. (1988). On-the-job back exercises. *American Journal of Nursing, 88*, 656-659.

Gramling, A. (1995). What's so new about demand management? *Managed Care, 4*, 4, 33-37.

Ham, F. (1989). How companies are making wellness a family affair. *Business and Health, 7*, 9, 33.

Hardy, A. et al. (1986). The economic impact of the first 10,000 cases of Acquired Immunodeficiency Syndrome in the United States. *Journal of the American Medical Association, 255*, 209.

Hilyer, J., Brown, K., Sirles, A. and Peoples, L. (1990). A flexibility intervention to reduce the incidence and severity of joint injuries among municipal fire fighters. *Journal of Occupational Medicine, 32*, 631-638.

Hospital's back injury prevention program cuts injuries, time lost, workmen's comp. (1995). *OSHA Week, 6*, 1 and 8.

Jackson, S., Chenoweth, D., Glover, E., White, D., and Chenier, T. (1989). Study indicates smoking cessation improves workplace absenteeism rate. *Occupational Health and Safety, 58,* 12, 13-18.

Jacobson, M. (1994). Compelling reasons for employers to invest in maternal and child health. *Presentation at the National Managed Health Care Summit*, Washington, D.C., April 12.

Kaman, R. (Ed.) 1995. *Worksite health promotion economics.* Champaign, IL: Human Kinetics Publishing.

Kandel, B. (1989, January 12). Controversy greets nation's 1st VDT law. *USA Today,* p. 3A.

Kemper, D. (1992). Should there be self-care in your corporation's cost-containment future? *Health Promotion Today.* Kalamazoo, MI: International Health Awareness Center, Inc.

Koplan, J., Powell, K., Sikes, R., Shirley, R., and Campbell, CC. (1985). An epidemiologic study of the benefits and risks of running. *Journal of the American Medical Association, 248,* 3118-3121.

Koplan, J., Siscovick, D., and Goldbaum, G. (1985). The risks of exercise: A public health view of injuries and hazards. *Public Health Reports, 100,* 189-195.

Kristein, M. (1983). How much can business expect to profit from smoking cessation? *Preventive Medicine, 12,* 358-381.

Kelsey, J. and Golden, A. (1987). Occupational and workplace factors associated with low back pain. *Occupational Medicine, 2,* 7-16.

Landgreen, M. (1990). Coca-Cola's back care program decreases accident rate by 83%. *Club Industry, 6,* 15.

Luce, B. and Schweitzer, S. (1978, March 9). Smoking and alcohol abuse: a comparison of their economic consequences. *New England Journal of Medicine,* 569-57.

Mauro, T. and Beissert, T. (1987, March 4). Court gives AIDS victims job support. *USA Today,* p. A1.

McDonald, M. (1990). How to deal with AIDS in the work place. *Business and Health, 8,* 7, 12-22.

Merritt, N. (1987, March 23). Bank of America's blueprint for a policy on AIDS. *BusinessWeek,* p. 127.

Metropolitan Insurance (1995). The urgency of visits to hospital emergency departments: data from the national hospital ambulatory medical care survey (NHAMCS). 1992 *Statistical Bulletin, 76,* 10-19.

Morris, A.(1984). Program compliance key to preventing low back injuries. *Occupational Health and Safety, 51,* 44-47.

Morris, A. (1984). Back rehabilitation programs speed recovery of injured workers. *Occupational Health and Safety, 53,* 7, 53-68.

Nathan, P., Keniston, R., Myers, L., and Meadows, K. (1992). Obesity as a risk factor for slowing of sensory conduction of the median nerve in industry. *Journal of Occupational Medicine, 4,* 379-382.

Healthy People 2000 at work: Strategies for employers. Appendix A. (1991). Washington, D.C.: National Resource Center on Worksite Health Promotion.

Painter, K. (1991, June 20). Cost of AIDS care: Sky-high and rising. *USA Today,* p. D6.

Shepherd, R.J. (1992). A critical analysis of work-site fitness programs and their postulated economic benefits. *Medicine and Science in Sports and Exercise, 24,* 354-370.

Shore, G., Prasad, P., and Zroback, M. (1989). Metrofit: a cost-effective fitness program. *Fitness in Business, 3,* 147-153.

Silverstein, B. and Armstrong, T. (1988). Can in-plant exercise control musculoskeletal symptoms? *Journal of Occupational Medicine, 30,* 922-927.

Sirles, A., Brown, K., and Hilyer, J.(1991). Effects of back school education and exercise in back injured municipal workers. *Journal of the American Association of Occupational Health Nursing, 39,* 7-12.

Spoth, R. (1991). Formative research on smoking cessation program attributes preferred by smokers. *American Journal of Health Promotion, 5,* 3, 346-354.

Stanforth, D. and Plattor, KJ. (1993). Implementing and evaluating a work station stretching program. *American Journal of Health Promotion, 7,* 73.

Stine, G.J. (1995). *AIDS update 1994-1995.* New York: Prentice-Hall.

Stress claims are making business jumpy. (1985, October 14). *BusinessWeek,* pp. 152-153.

Swerdlin, M. (1989). Investing in healthy babies pays off. *Business and Health, 7,* 7, 38-40.

Taravella, S. (1990, February 19). Self-insured employers limit AIDS benefits. *Modern Healthcare,* p. 52.

Terry, P. (1987). Finding the causes of back pain helps workers, companies recover. *Occupational Health and Safety, 56,* 8, 15-20.

Thompson, D.A. (1990). Effect of exercise breaks on musculoskeletal strain among data-entry operators: a case study. In *Promoting Health and Productivity in the Computerized Office* by Steven Saulter et al. Taylor and Francis Publishers.

Tsai, S., Bernacki, E., and Baun, W. (1988). Injury prevalence and associated costs among participants of an employee fitness program. *Preventive Medicine, 17,* 475-482.

Tsai, S., Gilstrap, E., Cowles, S., Waddell, L., and Ross, C. (1992).

Personal and job characteristics of musculoskeletal injuries in an industrial population. *Journal of Occupational Medicine, 34,* 606-611.

U. S. Department of Labor, Bureau of Labor Statistics. CTD incidence in American industry. Personal communication, February 1, 1993.

U.S. Department of Labor, Bureau of Labor Statistics. (1992). Newsletter, November 18, 1 and 11.

Van Camp, S.P. (1995). ACSM offers more than exercise lite. *Fitness Management, 11,* 18.

Van Tuinen, M. and Land, G. (1986). Smoking and excess sick leave in a department of health. *Journal of Occupational Medicine, 28,* 1, 33-35.

Vickery, D. and Fries, J. (1990). *Take care of yourself: Your personal guide to self-care and preventing illness.* 4th Edition. Reading, MA: Addison-Wesley Publishing Company.

Walker, C. (1991). Healthy babies for healthy companies. *Business and Health, 9,* 5, 29-30.

Walsh, D. (1984). Corporate smoking policies: a review and an analysis. *Journal of Occupational Medicine, 26,* 1, 17.

Walter, S., Sutton, J., and McIntosh, J. (1985). The aetiology of sports injuries: a review of methodologies. *Sports Medicine, 2,* 47-58.

Weis, W. (1981). Can you afford to hire smokers? *Personnel Administrator, 26,* 5, 71-78.

Whitmer, W. (1992, Mid-March). The city of Birmingham's wellness partnership contains medical costs. Business and Health, 60-66.

CHAPTER 7

AWHP Compensation and benefits survey (1993). Association for Worksite Health Promotion, Northbrook, IL.

Burke, R. and Robson, R. (1995). In and outsourcing: how to assess vendors. *AWHP's Worksite Health, 1,* 14-16.

Dimmitt, B. (1995). ADA: revealing the legal impact, shaping employer tactics. *Business and Health, 13,* 7, 27-34.

Employee self-decisions produce immediate health cost savings (1995). *Employee Benefit Plan Review, 49,* 12, 55.

Herbert, D. (1990). Suit against treadmill manufacturer dismissed. *Fitness Management, 6,* 2, 25.

Herbert, D. (1990). Health club release may not be valid. *Fitness Management, 6,* 5, 24.

Johnson, D. (1997). Renovation. *Fitness Management,* April 1997, 30-32.

Most HMOs provide health promotion services to members. (1995). *Employee Benefit Plan Review, 49,* 12, 56.

Pessin, F. (1995). Maximizing limited space. *Fitness Management, 11,* 10, 36-39.

Ritzer, J. (1990). Ten steps to follow when building/remodeling locker rooms. *Club Industry, 6,* 3, 25.

Sattler, T. and Donick, C. (1995). How to choose trouble-shooting consultants. *Fitness Management, 11,* 40-41.

Silveous, E. and Pfeiffer, G. (1995). Six Elements of a Successful Communication Strategy. *AWHP's Worksite Health, 2,* 3, 25-28.

Wood, B. (1986). The new aerobics floors. *Club Industry, 2,* 5, 23-25.

CHAPTER 8

Alexy, B. and Eynon, D. (1991). A strategy for health promotion at multiple worksites. *AAOHN Journal, 39,* 2, 53-56.

Bertera, R. (1991). The effects of behavioral risks on absenteeism and health care costs in the workplace. *Journal of Occupational Medicine, 33,* 11, 1119-1124.

Brink, S. (1987). *Health risks and behavior: The impact on medical costs.* Brookfield, WI: Milliman and Robertson, Inc.

DeJoy, D. and Southern, D. (1993). An integrated perspective on work-site health promotion. *Journal of Occupational Medicine, 35,* 12, 1221-1230.

Detert, R. and Kidd, T. (1989). Identifying the feasibility of health promotion at the small worksite. *Fitness in Business, 4,* 131-135.

Health Risks and Their Impact on Medical Costs. (1995). Brookfield, WI: Milliman and Robertson, Inc. and Staywell Health Management Systems, Inc. in conjunction with the Chrysler Corporation and the International Union, UAW.

Proschaska, J., Norcross, J., and DiClemente, C. (1994). *Changing for good.* New York: William Morrow and Company.

CHAPTER 9

Alexy, B. and Eynon, D. (1991). A strategy for health promotion at multiple corporation sites. *AAOHN Journal, 39,* 2.

Hersen, M., Eisler, R., and Miller, P. (1992). *Progress in behavior modification.* Sycamore Publishing Company, 1992.

Medrea, J. (1995). How Champion merged health and family services into its business plan. *AWHP's Worksite Health*, Winter, 32-35.

Prochaska, J., Norcross, J., and DiClemente, C. (1994). *Changing for Good*. William Morrow and Company, Inc.

Ramizez, S. (1994). *Health promotion for all: Strategies for reaching diverse populations at the workplace.* Wellness Councils of America.

CHAPTER 10

AWHP Professional Standards Task Force, (1995). How do you measure up? Guidelines for the worksite health promotion director. *AWHP's Worksite Health*, 2, 3, 18-23.

Check out these publications for your professional library. (1996) *AWHP's Worksite Health*, 3, 2, 18-19.

Chen, M. and Jones, R. (1982). Preparing health educators for the workplace: a university-health insurance company alliance. *Health Values*, 6, 6, 9-12.

Chenoweth, D. (1983). Health education in the private sector: preparing tomorrow's health management personnel. *Health Education, 14*, 3, 28-34.

Chenoweth, D. (1995). Health promotion in small businesses. Chapter 12 in *Critical Issues in Worksite Health Promotion*. Mark Wilson and David DeJoy (Eds.). Needham Heights, MA: Allyn and Bacon.

Cottrell, R. (1986). Curriculum guidelines studied. *AFB Region II Newsletter*, 2, 1, 2-3.

Cottrell, R. and Wagner, D. (1990). Internships in community health education/promotion: professional preparation programs. *Health Education, 20*, 1, 30-33.

Cottrell, R., Gutting, J., and Davis, L. (1990). Content priorities for training in health/fitness management: comparison of program directors and faculty members. *American Journal of Health Promotion, 4*, 5, 8-11.

DuBois, P. (1995). Certification: how to spot the real thing. *Fitness Management, 13*, 9, 46-48.

Golaszewski, T. (1981). Health education for corporations: efforts toward a professional preparation program. *Health Education, 12*, 6, 5.

Golaszewski, T. et al. (1982). Competency identification, evaluation and improvement for corporate health program fitness specialists: health education variables. *Health Education, 13*, 4, 32-35.

Gorman, D., Brown, B., and Di Brezzo, R. (1986). Professional training for corporate wellness personnel: survey results from practicing professionals. *Health Education, 17*, 5, 71-74.

Jones, J. and Ver Voort, G. What employers want: UWSP-AWHP survey results. Presentation at *1995 American Alliance for Health, Physical Education, Recreation and Dance Annual Convention*, Cincinnati, Ohio.

Sawyer, T. (1985). The employee program director, part 2: position and career path. *Corporate Fitness and Recreation*, October/November, 43-47.

Sawyer, T. (1986). The employee program director, part 3: visions of the year 2000. *Corporate Fitness and Recreation*, December/January, 43-50.

INDEX

health risks. *See also* health risk appraisal
   ailments associated with 21
   cost sharing of 9–10, 105
   costs per 10–11
   levels per number of factors 44
   modifiable lifestyle factors 10–11, 130
   most common 9, 89
   prospective medicine for 23
   requiring GXT protocol 46
health screening
   after several sessions 45
   classifications for 46
   for employer risk reduction 42, 46–47
   outsourcing of 108
   for planning 18, 44–45
   pre-exercise 45–48
   during pregnancy 98
   as primary prevention 13
   for small businesses 47–48, 129
   standards for 44
   techniques for 44–46
Healthworks 121
Healthy Employees Lifestyles Program (HELP) 155
Healthy People 2000 5, 102
heart disease
   as health risk 46, 92
   screening protocol for 44–46, 48
heart rate 50
helplessness 89
high blood pressure. *See* hypertension
high-risk employees
   attracting participation by 18, 60, 98
   EAPs for 85
   examples of 10–11
   identifying for referral 44
   in multi-site businesses 135
   placement in programs 55, 57
   in small businesses 130
   telephone counseling services for 105
HIV (Human Immunodeficiency Virus)
   economic cost of 102–103
   principles for worksites 103–104
   resources for 151–152
HMOs. *See* Health Maintenance Organizations
home remedies 105
honor system 59
housing assistance 85
HRA. *See* health risk appraisal
Human Resource departments
   data from 20
   integrating programs with 34, 38
   for policy changes 81
humidity 93
humor room 89
HVAC (heating, ventilating, and air conditioning system) 93
hyperglycemia. *See* diabetes mellitus
hyperlipidemia 45
hypertension
   as health risk 9, 11, 46
   programs for 49, 72, 105
hyperuricemia 45

I

ICD codes. *See* International Classification of Disease
IDEA, The Int'l Association of Fitness 166
identification phase 17–24
   for multi-site businesses 131–133
   for small businesses 129–130
identity protection. *See* confidentiality

illegal drug abuse. *See* substance abuse
image, company 6
immunizations 13
implementation phase 18–19, 53–64
   for multi-site businesses 133–136
   for small businesses 129
inactivity 21, 60
incentives. *See also* rewards
   external 58–59, 69, 95
   for high-risk employees 60, 69
   outsourcing implementation of 108
   for prenatal programs 98
incentive survey 26–28, 58
independent variables, in evaluation 69
indoor tracks 94
inflation 4, 7, 10
Informed Consent Forms 46–47
injuries, occupational. *See* occupational injuries
injuries, program-related. *See* liability risks
instructors. *See* specialists, health promotion and fitness
insurance pooling 129–130
integrated health management 34–35, 38–39
   model programs of 119–120, 123
   in multi-site businesses 138
interest, employee
   conflicts with needs 25–26, 28
   identification of 19–20, 60
interest, national 6
Interest Survey Form (ISF) 18, 24–26
International Classification of Disease (ICD) 20, 22
internships
   criteria for admission 146–147
   guidelines for 147
   opportunity sources 146
   requirements for 147–148
ISF. *See* Interest Survey Form

J

job interviews 149
job market
   opportunity sources 146
   professionally preparing for 144–149
   WHP's potential 143–144
jogging 80, 83, 94
Johnson & Johnson 12, 54
jute backing 93

K

Kimberly-Clark Corporation 5
Koop, C. Everett 103, 115, 119

L

lab tests, for screening 44–45
Langley Air Force Base 121–122
large businesses
   EAPs for 86
   personnel resources in 106–107
   task forces in 19
lawsuits. *See* liability risks
learning style 110
legal assistance
   for employees 85
   for employers 44, 46, 86, 101
Levi Strauss 103
liability insurance
   for equipment manufacturers 92
   for health care providers 7
   for interns 147
liability risks
   from allowing smoking 98–99, 101
   of EAP activity 86

ABOUT THE AUTHOR

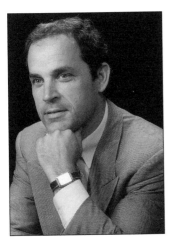

As a professor of health education and worksite health promotion studies at East Carolina University, David Chenoweth, PhD, FAWHP, has taught, advised, and counseled undergraduate and graduate students for 20 years; in the 10 years that he's directed the undergraduate worksite health promotion program, student enrollment has grown 800 percent.

Dr. Chenoweth also has nearly 20 years' professional consulting experience as president of Health Management Associates. He's made over 300 presentations to various business and health care groups and has authored five previous books on the subject, including *Planning Health Promotion at the Worksite* and *Health Care Cost Management*.

A fellow of the Association for Worksite Health Promotion (AWHP) and a member of the Wellness Councils of American (WELCOA), Dr. Chenoweth is the education/university chair for AWHP Region II, from which he received the President's Award in 1995. Since 1988 he has chaired the Business and Industry Committee of North Carolina's Council on Physical Fitness and Health. He was one of 11 nationwide authorities to serve on AWHP's economic impact panel in 1993, and he currently serves on a panel to evaluate WELCOA award applications.

Dr. Chenoweth received his PhD from The Ohio State University in 1980. He and his wife, Katie, and son, Zachary, live in New Bern, North Carolina. In his leisure time Dr. Chenoweth enjoys golf, tennis, biking, and landscaping.

ADDITIONAL WORKSITE HEALTH PROMOTION BOOKS

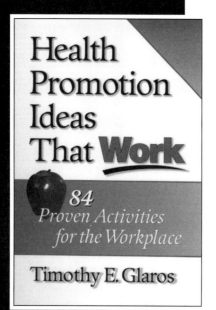

These 84 fresh, inexpensive, and easy-to-implement ideas are sure to boost participation and get results. Health promotion expert Timothy Glaros explains ways individuals coordinating worksite health promotions can concentrate on program implementation and maintenance without getting bogged down in the process of devising program concepts. Covering the full range of common health concerns and core program activities, this book features ideas for effective worksite promotions on numerous health topics and includes seasonal and holiday themes.

1997 • Paper • 152 pp • Item BGLA0888
ISBN 0-87322-888-X • $20.00 ($29.95 Canadian)

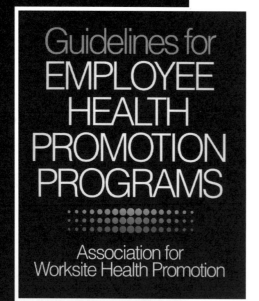

Developed by the Association for Worksite Health Promotion (AWHP), the premier organization for corporate health promotion professionals, this book guides you—step by step—through the phases of an employee health promotion initiative. It not only details the framework for designing a program tailored to your employee population and financial resources, but also sets 10 quality standards for a successful program. An essential resource for every business and health promotion professional concerned with corporate health promotion.

1992 • Paper • 152 pp • Item BAFB0351
ISBN 0-87322-351-9 • $29.00 ($43.50 Canadian)

HUMAN KINETICS
The Information Leader in Physical Activity
http://www.humankinetics.com/

For more information or to place your order, U.S. customers
call toll-free 1-800-747-4457.
Customers outside the U.S. use the appropriate
telephone number/address shown in the front of this book.

2335